NURSING OLDER PEOPLE

This practical guide helps student and practising nurses to understand the impact of their care when working with older people. With stories from older people who have had varied experiences of health care and nursing, chapters are underpinned by five key principles: providing patient-centered and dignified care, shared decision-making involving family and friends, multidisciplinary care, improving well-being through companionship and a sense of value, and an appreciation of both the challenges and rewards of working with older people.

This book offers:

- Stories which reflect the complexity of care and health experienced by older people and their journeys.
- Topic-oriented chapters which provide a series of evidence-based readings which use the most up-to-date research evidence merged with national and international policy and practitioner experience.
- Practical tips and key messages for working with older people.

The volume can be used to help nursing students and practising nurses to understand better how their care might impact positively on older people's health and well-being. This situates the reader within the world as experienced by older people.

Heather Fillmore Elbourne, RN, PhD, is a researcher, educator, and specialist in geriatric nursing. Her skills and expertise lie in clinical nursing, interdisciplinary geriatric education, and clinical decision-making. Her doctoral research focused on the interdisciplinary care of older adults and the implementation of Person-Centred Intermediate Care in the UK. Her subsequent research has concentrated on understanding better the impact of frailty in older age and the value of interdisciplinary care when striving to best meet the needs of older adults.

Andrée le May, RN, BSc, PhD, PGCE(A), is a nurse, teacher, and researcher. Her work focuses on how nurses use knowledge in practice, and whenever possible she combines this with her clinical specialism of elderly care. She is Professor Emerita at the University of Southampton and co-editor of the *Journal of Research in Nursing*.

NURSING OLDER PEOPLE

Realities of Practice

Edited by Heather Fillmore Elbourne
and Andrée le May

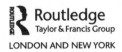

Routledge
Taylor & Francis Group

LONDON AND NEW YORK

First published 2020
by Routledge
2 Park Square, Milton Park, Abingdon, Oxon OX14 4RN

and by Routledge
52 Vanderbilt Avenue, New York, NY 10017

Routledge is an imprint of the Taylor & Francis Group, an informa business

British Library Cataloguing-in-Publication Data
A catalogue record for this book is available from the British Library

Library of Congress Cataloging-in-Publication Data
Names: Elbourne, Heather, editor. | le May, Andrée, editor.
Title: Nursing older people: realities of practice / [edited by] Heather Elbourne and Andrée le May. Other titles: Nursing older people (Elbourne)
Description: Abingdon, Oxon; New York, NY: Routledge, 2019. |
Includes bibliographical references and index.
Identifiers: LCCN 2018060075 | ISBN 9781498735179 (pbk.) |
ISBN 9781315116129 (e-book)
Subjects: | MESH: Geriatric Nursing—methods | Aged—psychology |
Aging Classification: LCC RC954 | NLM WY 152 | DDC 618.97/0231—dc23
LC record available at https://lccn.loc.gov/2018060075

ISBN: 978-0-367-33143-6 (hbk)
ISBN: 978-1-4987-3517-9 (pbk)
ISBN: 978-1-315-11612-9 (ebk)

Typeset in Interstate
by codeMantra

CONTENTS

CONTRIBUTORS

Imogen Blood is a qualified social worker, with 20 years' experience of research, policy, and service development with and for older people and those living with dementia. As Director of Imogen Blood & Associates Ltd since 2009, she has written about and trained health- and social-care professionals on 'positive risk'. (Imogen@imogenblood.co.uk)

Heather Fillmore Elbourne is a nurse, researcher, teacher and specialist in interdisciplinary approaches to geriatric care. Her skills and expertise lie in clinical nursing, nursing education, and interdisciplinary clinical decision-making. Her doctoral research focused on the interdisciplinary approach to implementation of Person-Centred Intermediate Care in the United Kingdom. Her subsequent research concentrates on understanding better the impact of frailty in older age and the need for interdisciplinary collaboration and care. (heather.elbourne@gmail.com)

Catherine Evans is a HEE/NIHR Senior Clinical Lecturer and Honorary Nurse Consultant in Palliative Care. Catherine's research and clinical practice concerns developing and evaluating palliative and community-care services and interventions for older people living with frailty and multimorbidity. She focuses on the integration of palliative and geriatric care. (catherine.evans@kcl.ac.uk)

Khim Horton is an Independent Consultant in Care of Older People. She is a nurse by profession and has spent much of her career working in higher education as a researcher and teacher. Now a Visiting Senior Lecturer, City University of London, Khim continues to work closely with the Royal College of Physicians on inpatient falls audits. (khim.horton@gmail.com)

Andrée le May is a nurse, teacher, and researcher. Her work focuses on how nurses use knowledge in practice, and whenever possible she combines this with her clinical specialism of elderly care. She is Professor Emerita at the University of Southampton and co-editor of the Journal of Research in Nursing. (aclm@soton.ac.uk)

Caroline Nicholson is a clinical academic nurse. Her research programme and clinical practice focus on the intersection between gerontological and end-of-life care. She is interested in the capabilities and frailties of older people and the development of care systems to promote quality at end of life. (caroline.nicholson@kcl.ac.uk)

Ken Rockwood is a Professor of Medicine (geriatric medicine and neurology) at Dalhousie University, Canada, and an active staff physician at the Queen Elizabeth II Health Sciences Centre in Halifax, Nova Scotia. He is a leading authority on frailty and has researched, taught, and published widely in this field. (Kenneth.Rockwood@Dal.Ca)

Samuel Searle is a geriatrician based in Canada. His academic training was in the United States, Canada, and the United Kingdom. He is currently pursuing a PhD at University College London on frailty in the acute care setting by the grace of his wife Amy and their Labrador retriever. (samuelsearle@gmail.com)

ACKNOWLEDGEMENTS

In addition to chapter authors four people have made particular contributions to this book and we would like to thank them. They have helped us bring the realities of practice to these pages.

Nick Andrews, Research and Practice Development Officer, Wales School for Social Care Research, University of Swansea. (n.d.andrews@swansea.ac.uk)

Natasha Duke, Nurse Practitioner and part-time doctoral student at the University of Southampton. (N.Duke@soton.ac.uk)

Michelle Howarth, Senior Lecturer in the School of Health and Society at the University of Salford. (m.l.howarth2@salford.ac.uk)

Jenni Lynch, Early Career Research Fellow in the Centre for Research into Primary and Community Care at the University of Hertfordshire. (j.lynch5@herts.ac.uk)

1   About this book

Andrée le May and Heather Fillmore Elbourne

This book is guided by the following principles:

- Older people should receive dignified care; in order to do this care must centre around the person.
- Families and friends need to be included in care and care decisions to minimise isolation either of the older person or of the family member/friend.
- Older people require care from multidisciplinary teams, and nurses need to form an integral part of these teams.
- Companionship and feeling valued can increase feelings of mental well-being, and these are important parts of nursing care.
- Nursing older people can be challenging but also vastly rewarding.

Our aim is to help nursing students and practising nurses to understand better how their care might impact positively on older people's health and well-being. To do this, we have decided to first situate the reader within the world as experienced by older people by describing key facts about the ageing population, their health, and nursing (Chapter 2) and telling some stories based on older people's experiences of health and social care (Chapter 3). We believe that this approach will make it easier for readers to understand the impact of nursing and how nursing can be best structured if nurses start from the client's and their family's perspectives. Stories are a powerful way of showing what life is like for people in different circumstances, and we use them in the remaining chapters to develop empathy and understanding related to clinical situations. We have deliberately chosen stories that focus on the common difficulties of older age and emphasise that nurses form part of a team of health- and social-care workers.

One of the greatest fears expressed by older people is what will happen to them as they become functionally, physically, mentally, and/or socially more dependent on others as they grow frailer and less able to do the things they used to do. For many older people, and their families, friends, and carers, this change in independence brings with it unfamiliar risks and challenges. Understanding and managing such risks may be one of the most daunting aspects of ensuring that care is truly person-centred and works for the benefit of each individual person. In Chapter 4 Imogen Blood explores risk taking and risk management. We have deliberately situated this chapter early in the book since we believe that understanding and managing risk sensitively is crucial to the provision of high-quality care and the promotion of increased quality of life.

This book is not a comprehensive textbook of elderly care/geriatric nursing; rather we have picked commonly occurring consequences of the ageing process to explore how nurses might provide evidence-based, person-centred, responsive care to older people in these circumstances. In Chapter 5 we focus on the notion of staying healthy in older age by covering topics such as exercise, mental agility, and social interaction. This is complemented by Chapter 6 where Khim Horton focuses on common difficulties experienced by older people including falling, incontinence, loneliness, and pain. In Chapter 7 Samuel Searle and Ken Rockwood discuss frailty as an independent geriatric condition that includes both physical and psychological decline and too often goes unnoticed as symptoms are attributed to the ageing process. This chapter is essential to nurses as the ability to identify frailty in its early stages is key to developing specific interventions that may delay or prevent further functional decline and other negative outcomes—such as acute illness, falls, hospitalisation, and death. Catherine Evans and Caroline Nicholson discuss end-of-life care in Chapter 8 making the critical point that dying and death are integral components of living in older age.

In these issue-specific chapters (4-8) experts have provided evidence-based readings using the most up-to-date research evidence merged with national and international policy and practitioner experience to highlight the best practice that a nurse can deliver in conjunction with the patient, their family, and the multidisciplinary/multi-agency team. We have deliberately used a blend of evidence sources—from patients, families, and clients; from the research literature; from policy directives and clinical guidelines, and from best practice and education to reflect the ways through which practitioners learn and function. Our thoughts on what comprises good practice are based on the concept of 'mindlines' (Gabbay and le May, 2004, 2011)—internalised, multiple sources of evidence, which are collectively reinforced, partly tacit, guidelines-in-the-head that clinicians use to flexibly guide and develop their practice.

We conclude in Chapter 9 by drawing together key points from the previous chapters which we believe will help nurses to understand better how their care might impact positively on older people's health and well-being.

References

Gabbay J and le May A (2004) Evidence-based guidelines or collectively constructed "mindlines"? An ethnographic study of knowledge management in primary care. *British Medical Journal* 329 (October 30) 1013-20.

Gabbay J and le May A (2011) *Practice-Based Evidence for Healthcare: Clinical Mindlines*. Routledge, Abingdon.

2 Thinking about the ageing population

Heather Fillmore Elbourne and Andrée le May

Introduction

As more and more people live longer their chances of needing care increase. There are several reasons for this which largely focus on the individual older person, their lay carers/ families, and/or their environmental/social circumstances. An older person may need more care when acutely ill than they did when they were younger; or they may be generally frailer in older age and need more help and support with activities of living and staying physically and mentally well; or they may not have familial or social support readily available; or they may be living with long-term, often multiple conditions that require continuing care and support. Each of these circumstances, taken individually or together, will impact on a person's physical and mental wellness.

Knowing more about ageing and its impact can help nurses to positively affect the health and wellness of older people (Andrews et al. 2015, Nunnelee et al. 2015), so before we think more about providing care and support to this group there are a few key facts that we need to consider. First, changing demographics means that there are more older people than ever before in almost every country in the world—older people are the fastest growing demographic cohort in the world (WHO 2015a). Second, older people are not only living longer, but they are also living longer with more complex health- and social-care needs (Wolff et al. 2002, Abellan van Kan et al. 2010, Rockwood and Mitnitski 2011). Third, there is both subtle and blatant ageism around us all in our work and everyday lives, and nurses need to understand how that might impact on older people and their care and how to minimise or, preferably, erase ageism by challenging negative stereotypes (Martin et al. 2009, Officer et al. 2016). Fourth, increased numbers of older people, with more complex health- and social-care needs, require increased levels of skilled nursing care; however, finding such nurses in sufficient quantities is becoming increasingly challenging. This chapter is largely about these four things.

Population ageing

Worldwide our population is ageing at an unprecedented rate. Globally, there is an increasing number of older adults alive, and they are living longer than at any other time in the history of humankind (Rechel et al. 2009, WHO 2017). Evidence from the World Health Organization (WHO 2009a) tells us that, on average, most people can expect to be alive and healthy into

---

Box 2.1 Some population facts (WHO 2009a, WHO 2015b, 2017)

The world's population is growing and ageing:

- Between 2000 and 2015 global life expectancy rose by five years–this is the fastest rise in human lifespans since the 1960s.
- Globally average life expectancy is 71.2 years. For women, it is 73.8 years, and for men, it is 69.1 years.
- Actual life expectancy varies amongst adults and countries, with Japan having the most extended lifespan at 84 years and Africa having the shortest life expectancy of 50 years (although this is increasing).

Simultaneously, at the opposite end of life:

- Fertility rates have declined in most countries around the world due to social changes such as the emancipation of women, growing economic prosperity, the availability of birth control, medical advancements, and public health campaigns.
- Worldwide, although a minority of nations have increasing fertility rates, globally fewer babies are being born.

---

their 60s and beyond (Box 2.1). Our global population is ageing *and* growing due to a reduction in global death rates and birth rates: this has social, health, and economic consequences that we have not faced before.

Whilst the significant increase in life expectancy means that there has been an overall improvement in health and living conditions around the world it brings with it several challenges for those involved in making health- and social-care policy and delivering care.

'Population Ageing' has become a standard idiom of our time and refers to the entire population growing older. Unlike individual people who age with each passing birthday, populations age when the percentage of young people in the population is less than the percentage of older adults in the population i.e. when fewer children are born than there are adults alive. Population ageing results in:

1   an increasing number of older people in our societies;
2   a reduction in the proportion of children;
3   a decline in the proportion of people of working age (~16–60 years) who can support those who do not work (WHO 2009a).

This demographic shift influences many of our societal, moral, and economic trends. For instance, it is unlikely that the increased numbers of older adults needing care and support will be matched by an adequate increase in the amount of resources (financial and human) that are available for this group to use (Kingma 2007, World Health Assembly 2011, Humphries et al. 2012, Nuernberger et al. 2018). Any shortage of working-aged, tax-paying adults is likely to result in less public money to support care *and* means that there will be fewer people to provide that care either in paid or in voluntary employment. This may be compounded by the reduction of familial care associated with the break-up of the nuclear family, easier national and international migration resulting in increased geographical distances between family members and less informal social support within communities (World Health Assembly 2011, Abhicharttibutra et al. 2017). These population changes and their resultant challenges have been building steadily since the post-World War II baby boom ended in the late 1960s (Butler 1969, WHO 2011, Beard et al. 2016) and are unlikely to change barring any unexpected or catastrophic occurrence. Meeting these challenges requires widespread progress in redefining and constructing health- and social-care systems to meet the complex needs of this group of people (Abhicharttibutra et al. 2017, Blood 2013, Buchan et al. 2015)–a group of people that spans 40 years and the various experiences and norms of those four different decades: for instance, the experiences and needs of the oldest old will be very different to those of the latest generation to enter older age–the baby boomers (see below).

Think about this ...

Economics is important!
Conceivably one of the driving forces behind increased attention to older people is that the latest generation to enter older age have money to spend! In general, the baby-boomers are entering their senior years financially stable with disposable income, thus resulting in an unprecedented, vast and relatively untapped market. Perhaps this is why stakeholders (peripheral to those attentive to health- and social-care service needs) e.g. in the field of commerce, appear to have quickly accepted the burgeoning importance of the increasing number of older people in our societies and have swiftly adapted to target this group as consumers from increasing attention to leisure opportunities to capitalising on life-style improvements. Next time you go to newsagents check out the magazines targeting older people you can see on the shelves. Flick through them and see what articles and features there are.

However, we remain ill-prepared to meet the needs and demands of what will quickly become one of the world's new population 'norms'(Marengoni et al. 2011, Conference Board of Canada 2013, Elbourne et al. 2013, Hominick et al. 2016) (see Preparing for the "Big Day").

Think about this ... Preparing for the "Big Day"

For a moment think about the following analogy:

The lack of preparation, and thus the situation older adults and those in health-and social-care services currently find themselves in might be equated to an all too familiar scenario. Pick your favourite yearly event or holiday i.e. a national holiday, Christmas, Hanukkah, Kwanzaa - any event that requires some forethought and planning. Now think about the day prior to that event and picture the scenario in which some people fill the shops on the eve of the holiday scrambling to purchase the perfect present or celebratory food, and find themselves left thinking "Wow how did this happen, it has just snuck up on me?!". Well, it did not! We all knew it was coming. It happens at the same time every year and thanks to our calendars and perhaps advertising we've been reminded continuously for weeks that the countdown to the event was on. Inevitably, there are always those left in a tizzy and scrambling at the last moment. Yet, there should be no shock, and the lack of preparedness should be solely planted on the shoulders of the person who is alone and manic in the shops as we all knew it was coming.

Here is where the comparison of being 'unprepared for something we all knew was coming' ends. Being unprepared for a holiday or yearly event will only result in the minor annoyance of having to endure a few hours of uncomfortable manic preparation. Whereas failure to prepare for the population change that we are experiencing is a completely different matter leaving contemporary health- and social-care services in a position that cannot be quickly or smoothly rectified and results in older adults receiving substandard care which could negatively affect the rest of their lives.

If you were a policy-maker what would you do? If you were an older person what would you do? If you belonged to a group advocating for older people what would you do?

Defining older age and older people's needs

Many people, when asked, can identify a point in time when they decide for themselves that they have reached older age—it could be retirement age, stopping work, having grandchildren, or simply feeling less (or more!) energetic. In addition to our personal definitions of old age there are societal definitions that tend to focus on laws and conventions and may change from time to time. For instance, as we write this book the retirement age in many high-income countries is 65 years but set to rise to 67 years in future; however, having a set age for retirement is a much rarer thing in some middle- to low-income countries. Some services such as health- and social-care services distinguish age into further classifications; for instance, health- and social-care services often divide older age into three discrete categories: old age (75–84), old-old age (85–94), and oldest-old age (95+). Doing this might seem slightly strange when other definitions start around the late 60s but this is one way to ensure that services and skilled teams are targeted to meet the increasingly more complex physiological, cognitive, and social needs of older people.

Whilst many older people need minimal care from health- and social-care services, others will have "high support needs" and as such require more intensive or prolonged care—some of which will rely either solely or partly on nurses. The Joseph Rowntree Foundation (JRF) defines older people who have high support needs as:

> Older people of any age who need a lot of support due to physical frailty, chronic conditions and/or multiple impairments (including dementia). Most will be over 85 years old, though some will be younger. Many will be affected by other factors including poverty,

disadvantage, nationality, ethnicity, lifestyle etc. Some of the very oldest people may never come into this category.

(Blood et al. 2010, p. 3)

All nurses whether they are qualified or students, specialists in elderly care or general adult, or mental health nurses will care for or provide advice to or about older people at some time in their careers. This inevitability means that all nurses must understand the effect of having high support needs on an older person and their family if they are to provide sound care.

Health and the ageing population

As we have seen living longer does not necessarily equate with living longer in good health, quantity of years does not directly correlate with quality of life. Recent evidence indicates there is a significant difference between a person's life expectancy and their healthy life expectancy– roughly seven/eight years (WHO 2011, Dewar and Nolan 2013). For those specifically concerned with health and human services this translates to hundreds of thousands of older people needing care and support towards the end of their lives. And these numbers will increase over the next 30 years or so. Experts predict, by the year 2050, one out of every five people will be 60 years of age or older. Additionally, those who live to the age of 85 can further expect to live around another seven years. Although those living the longest are unlikely to experience good health for all seven of those extra years: this group is projected to double in size to nearly 2 billion people–making it the fastest growing demographic group in the world (WHO 2015a).

It is clear then that there is a pressing need for change if we are to meet the health- and social-care needs and demands of the ageing population. Some of this modification needs to come from finding out the best ways to address the issues and challenges faced by older people, and this requires age-sensitive/relevant research that is multidisciplinary, multinational, and representative of the diversity that exists within present and future cohorts of older people (Conference Board of Canada 2013, WHO 2013a, b, 2015c, Bähler et al. 2015, Gould et al. 2015). The findings from this body of research need to underpin clinical practice, public health interventions, and health and social policies. Whilst age-appropriate, person-centred care is built on having the best evidence for care it is also about having adequate resources (including people with non-ageist views) to maintain the dignity and respect of those involved.

As the population ages and grows so too will the number of people living with chronic disease (Boyd et al. 2005, Rockwood et al. 2005, WHO 2009b, Bähler et al. 2015). Internationally, chronic long-term diseases now surpass infectious diseases as the leading cause of death and disability. Non-communicable diseases account for 46% of the worldwide burden of illness and 59% of the world's annual deaths (averaging 57 million) (WHO 2013a, 2015c)

Although older people experience acute illness and infections many older people have chronic, multiple, interacting health- and social-care needs that require sophisticated management by health- and social-care providers (Hoffman et al. 1996, Paez et al. 2009, Rechel et al. 2009, Elbourne et al. 2013, Oostrom et al. 2014). For most older people these long-term conditions are well-controlled and require little more than regular monitoring meetings with primary-care nurses and doctors, but for some people their conditions require more intensive care in hospitals or ongoing care at home or in residential or specialist nursing homes. Any older person, even after a short hospital stay for treatment of an acute condition, may lack the necessary financial/personal support needed to return home and have to remain longer in institutional care than needed. Older people require systems that can deal with their complex needs in an integrated way that promotes continuity and completeness of care (Wolff et al. 2002, Rechel et al. 2009, Steis et al. 2012, Fillmore Elbourne and le May 2015, Canadian Institute for Health Information 2016, Prentice et al. 2017).

Whilst older patients' needs and circumstances have changed significantly over the last few decades the systems developed to care for them have often not kept pace and require significant adjustment if they are to provide effective care. Older people with an acute, long-term, or palliative condition often require a multidisciplinary approach which can cut across the boundaries of health and social care (Elbourne et al. 2013, Fillmore Elbourne and le May 2015). But current demands frequently see those providing care struggling to deliver it because of staff shortages, bed shortages, seasonal pressures, and ineffective communications across departments or sectors, or simply because care is provided at a distance from supporting family and friends. However, not all change requires money or change to infrastructures. An example of this is the practical guide to care that resulted from the JRF's 5-year programme, A Better Life. The programme posed the question, "What needs to happen to make life better for older people who need a lot of support – now and in the future?" Many qualitative and quantitative research reports came from this programme and of specific note here is the practical guide for people working with older adults (Blood 2013). In this guide Blood and her colleagues set out seven challenges for care providers as well as numerous practical ideas as to how one could convert these into reality (Box 2.2). The seven challenges are central to the principles underpinning this book (see Chapter 1).

Box 2.2 The seven challenges set out in A Better Life (Blood, 2013, p. 13)

"We all need positive images and balanced narratives to challenge ageist assumptions. Old age is not about 'them', it is about all of us.

We all need to make the effort to see and hear the individual behind the label or diagnosis, taking into account the increasing diversity of older people as a demographic group.

We must ensure that all support is founded in, and reflects, meaningful and rewarding relationships. Connecting with others is a fundamental human need, whatever our age or support needs.

We need to use the many assets, strengths, and resources of older people with high support needs through recognising and creating opportunities for them to both give and receive support.

We must all be treated as citizens: equal stakeholders with both rights and responsibilities, not only as passive recipients of care. We must also have clarity on what we can reasonably expect from publicly funded services and what we will need to take responsibility for ourselves.

The individual and collective voices of older people with high support needs should be heard and given power. We must use a much wider range of approaches to enable this.

We need to be open to radical and innovative approaches; but we also need to consider how, often simple, changes can improve lives within existing models".

All too often the emphasis remains on the physical aspects of illness and recovery and fails to consider the impact that psychological health can have on an older person's wellness and independence. There is considerable evidence which shows that for older adults, psychological wellness decreases their need for health care and increases their quality of life (Prohaska et al. 2006, Worsfold 2013). Psychological *and* physical care are essential components of skilled nursing care, and we will come back to talk about this in subsequent chapters.

Regardless of age, patients are best served when they receive age-specific support and care (Mezey et al. 2004, Dewar and Nolan 2013, Dewar and Kennedy 2016, Hirst and Lane 2016, Melillo 2017) which reflects appropriate age-related policies and care practices. These should always show respect for the older person's human rights and freedoms; empower and enable older people and their families to be assertive and actively involved in their care; and ensure that health and social support focuses on maintaining and maximising independence whilst sensitively assessing risk. All care, from the policies set in the boardroom to care provided at the bedside, must be non-discriminatory.

Whilst we can each imagine the impact of increasing frailty and/or multimorbidity it is better to understand what older people themselves experience and so we have laid out short stories and examples throughout this book to help with this. In addition to reading these, consider asking older people and their families themselves about their experiences. JRF asked a team of researchers (Katz et al, 2011) to ask older people with high support needs what they valued in their lives and devised a wheel-shaped model to help portray these findings—you might consider using the areas covered in it to guide conversations with older people and their families. The model has at its centre the older person, they are surrounded by two circles—an outer circle and an inner circle. The outer circle focuses on what the person values—these are categorised as social, physical, and psychological factors. The social factors comprise cultural activities, making a contribution, social interaction, good relationships with carers, and personal relationships; the physical factors are getting out and about, physical health, physical activities, good environment, safety, and security; and the psychological factors are associated with mental health, sense of self, self-determination, continuity and adjusting to change, and humour and pleasure. The inner circle details factors that help the person to achieve or prevents them from achieving what they want from life (transport, equipment, technology, finances, information, support, and other people's time).

Using this sort of model in daily care can enable nurses to understand the person they are caring for better, to help build connections between everyone involved in care, and to tailor dignified care more appropriately to suit the older person and their family's needs. When you read the subsequent chapters of this book remember to think about Katz et al.'s model and compare your experiences in practice with these ideas. You will probably find that you need to expand the factors to suit the context of care that you are working in and each older person's individual wishes.

Several researchers have highlighted the importance of nurses building respectful relationships with older people and their carers/families to help to include them in decision-making, give them more control over their environments and care, and enable them to feel dignified and be heard (e.g. Bridges and Nugus 2010, Calnan et al. 2013, Andrews et al. 2015). Building such relationships is a cornerstone of good practice.

Think about this ...

Think back over your last year of work and build a picture of a person you've care for who has had high support needs and needed care either in hospital, a nursing or residential home or their own home. What were their needs and what did you and the other members of the multidisciplinary care team do to ensure that their care was person-centred and your relationships respectful? As you read through this book keep this person (and their family and carers) in your mind – how do they compare to the people in the stories used in later chapters?

Ageism

Many of you reading this chapter will have heard people talk about the "Silver Tsunami" metaphor. It is one of the most commonly used analogies associated with population ageing and is overtly ageist. The metaphor (with occasional variations e.g. "Gray/Grey Tsunami", the "Senior Tsunami", "Senior Wave") initially made its debut in the late 1980s (Barusch 2013), suggesting that population ageing could be as devastating to our world as a seismic sea wave is to a seaside community. Rather than water the "silver tsunami" has been described by some as bringing a 'wave' of dependent, chronically ill older adults that will flood health- and social-care systems, destroy our economies, and wash away the quality of life as we know it (Charise 2012). Such talk is obviously offensive and ageist.

Just like other "isms" (such as racism and sexism) the uses of the Silver Tsunami metaphor push forward an ageist agenda based on partial truths and designed to generate fear (Charise 2012). These partial truths include the fact that population ageing will result in the largest group of seniors our world has ever had and so could be used to justify the very large wave notion by some people: but that is where the comparison ends. Historic data indicates this demographic ratio has been in the making for the last four to five decades so ironically, the mere fact that the Silver Tsunami metaphor has been in circulation since the late 1980s shows that its arrival cannot be, as a tsunami, unexpected. The continued use of this metaphor and similar ones, such as military metaphors that focus on "fighting/ battling against old age', extends the fatalistic and negative perceptions of what it truly means to be an older person (Officer et al. 2016).

Box 2.3 An example of ageist talk

Such was the case when, a highly respected, trailblazing gerontology nurse in a position of authority joined in on an informal discussion I was having with a nursing student. The area in which we sat was an open concept nursing station, in the centre of a busy medical/surgical unit. At the time of the discussion, the unit's beds were predominantly filled by older people. The hallway adjacent to the nursing station was a flurry of family members, patients, and hospital staff. Busy professionals and students filled the seats close to us. The nursing student and I were discussing population ageing and the potential challenges that lay ahead for acute-care settings. Using a tone and volume that made the following comment easily heard, the gerontology nurse said, "All we hear about is how the grey tsunami is coming. The tsunami is not developing – it is here, and we are swimming in it as we speak!".

It is important that nurses fight ageism and set a positive example to others (Butler 1969, Haight et al. 1994, Herdman 2002, Ferrario et al. 2007, Martin et al. 2009). This starts with holding non-ageist attitudes and beliefs and ensuring that these are translated into everyday actions and conversations. Many people believe that they do not use ageist language, and only, when probed further with examples of ageist jargon, do they become aware of the extent of their habitual use of ageist language (see Box 2.3 for an example from HFE's personal experience).

Think about this ...

If this happened to you, what would your response be? Would your answers differ if you were:

- o   One of the patients on this unit?
- o   A family member of a person who is 79 years old and critically ill next to the nursing station?
- o   The senior medical doctor at the station beside the nurse?
- o   An administrator who just happened to walk in and hear this comment?

Take another minute to think some more:

Did the way you responded change depending on which person you were thinking of? If so, why? If not, why not?

A movement is now underway calling for the elimination of the 'Silver Tsunami' metaphor (and its variations). Critics of this metaphor are urging professionals to remove it in favour of 'neutral' language to describe population ageing (Martin et al. 2009, Charise 2012). Arguing that the unconscious use of ageist expressions, mainly by those genuinely interested in the quality of care and life for older adults (such as providers, professionals, policymakers, and practitioners), is one more telling sign of how far-reaching and ingrained ageism is (Butler 1969, 2002, Herdman 2002, de la Rue 2003, Gould et al. 2012).

In the case of the gerontology nurse referred to in Box 2.3 when engaging others in a conversation, we must be consciously aware of what is said, and the language used to convey this message. Because ageism is commonplace, many of us may not fully understand the extent to which ageism has permeated our language. Self-awareness is our professional responsibility, and to help us there is an increasing number of articles, podcasts, and books focused on putting a stop to ageism. It is important for us all to constantly model the way we would like others to be and remember that 'you must be the change you want to see in the world' (often attributed to Mahatma Gandhi).

Ageism doesn't only occur in conversations between people, it occurs in the media and in political and policy decisions at all levels. Worldwide, there is an increasing number of governments and world-class health- and social-care organisations that are calling for change. It is imperative that such change results in recognition and elimination of any obstinate institutionalised ageism that has permeated health- and social-care systems. Change that begins with the universal understanding that ageing and being old is not a disease to cure, or an issue to fix, or a problem to avoid but a challenge to be grasped with enthusiasm and creativity.

The nursing workforce

Advancements in medicine and technology have resulted in many older adults living longer, and with different health problems, to their ancestors. These advancements have resulted in a slow, yet steady, increase in the number of patients living with and needing care for long-term conditions, and, as a result of this, a change to the requirements of the workforce needed to care for them. The presence of, sometimes, multiple long-term conditions with their related multimorbidities is one of the determinants of the need for nursing and other forms of health care (WHO 2013a). As an example of this, let us look at two pieces of research–the first is the 2013 report from the Conference Board of Canada (CBC). In this report, the CBC estimates that by 2026, over 2.4 million Canadians aged 65+ will require continuing care support for chronic illness and by 2046, that number will reach nearly 3.3 million (The Conference Board of Canada 2013). In the second piece of work a Canadian research team noted that 81% of seniors who were living independently in the community had at least one chronic illness (Gould et al. 2012). Similarly, south of the Canadian border, in the United States of America, 88% of the US population aged 65+ have at least one chronic condition, and more than 75% of all US health-care expenditure is related to the treatment of chronic conditions (Wolff et al. 2002). These North American statistics closely mirror those found in other countries across the world (WHO 2015a, WHO 2017).

Changing demographics and disease profiles have a direct impact on many (if not all) health and social policies including workforce, this is particularly so for nurses who make up a significant portion of all health-care providers. For instance, in Canada, regulated nurses comprise 48% of all health-care professionals (Canadian Institute for Health Information (CIHI) 2011). This ratio of nurses to all other health-care professionals is similar around the world. As such, globally, the demand for nurses is tremendous and is predicted to increase exponentially as the population continues to age and the prevalence of those living with chronic conditions increases (Wolff et al. 2002, CIHI 2010, 2011, Gould et al. 2012, Royal

College of Nursing (RCN) 2017). In response to this, governments and policymakers have begun to set out changes to their health- and social-care systems in order to meet the increasing needs of their ageing societies (Fillmore Elbourne and le May 2015, Humphries 2015, Oliver 2018).

However, despite this attention the lack of services and, sometimes, misuse of those we have can create workforce—or skills shortages. The lack of available nurses is compounded by environmental and geographical factors e.g. rurality and remoteness, where recruitment and retention of health professionals has historically been challenging (Rechel et al. 2009a, Gould et al. 2012). Rural health and providing the workforce required in such geographical areas is a worldwide challenge. Reports tell us that specifically, within Canada for instance, the overall demand for nurses to provide continuing care to older people in the community alone will increase from just under the current 64,000 in full-time jobs to 142,000 full-time jobs by 2035. This demand equates to an annual growth rate of 3.4% in community nursing; however, this demand shows no sign of being met by a growth in the supply (or retention) of nurses (O'Brien-Pallas et al. 2010, Canada 2017). A similar picture, relating to the entire nursing workforce, frequently makes the headlines in the United Kingdom.

Be it in Canada, the United Kingdom, or anywhere else in the world, be it in community health, home care, acute care, or long-term residential care, nursing shortages have reached hazardous levels. This problematic situation has led to many nurses working, all too often, at a near-crisis level (Bähler et al. 2015, Oliver 2018). In addition to critical staffing conditions in both rural and urban settings, many high-income countries are struggling with inadequate social support, rehabilitation services, and insufficient long-term and residential-care beds to meet the current needs of older adults: let alone the forecasted demands of population ageing (Rechel et al. 2009, WHO 2009b).

What about the future?

We need to consider what will be the overall effect of population ageing on our existing health- and social-care structures—will it be antagonistic or affable? Will population ageing overwhelm current health- and social-care systems, or will it enrich lives and communities, while laying a progressive age-friendly blueprint for generations to come? There are people on both sides of the divide who continue to build evidence supporting their claims, but we can be certain that the result, as well as any outcomes along the way, will directly correlate to the manner in which governments, administrators, policymakers, educators, and practitioners (to name a few) respond to population ageing.

Up until recently, the education nurses received was structured predominantly around the otherwise healthy individual experiencing an acute phase of illness or injury. Whilst this type of nursing remains necessary, it is clear that most older people will need a different sort of care—care which focuses on the intricacies of the ageing process and the synergistic effects that multiple chronic illnesses can have on an older person and their family. In order to cater for such complex needs nursing has to be more person-centred than ever before (Mezey et al. 2004, Krichbaum et al. 2015, Hirst and Lane 2016) as well as being flexible enough to cater for a myriad of needs from maintaining wellness, through illness to death. Nurses need to have a sophisticated understanding of and confidence in managing common frailty syndromes such as dementia and falls, managing complex changes in levels of dependency and care needs which result in loss of function and independence, and recognising and managing often subtly deteriorating conditions as well as issues such as safeguarding in older people.

It is the responsibility of the professionals caring for older people and their families to ensure there are sufficient highly skilled nurses, working in multidisciplinary, multi-agency teams, having access to and using the best evidence to provide care that best meets older people's changing and complex needs. Being educated and competent in the intricacies of geriatrics/elderly care is no longer an issue of professional choice. It is an issue of patient safety and ethical responsibility for most practising nurses. We hope this book enables you to feel more confident in caring for older people in whatever setting you are working in.

Summary of key messages

- Changing demographics means that there are more older people than ever before in almost every country in the world—older people are the fastest growing demographic cohort in the world.
- Older people are not only living longer but they are living longer with more complex health- and social-care needs.
- There is both subtle and blatant ageism around us all in our work and everyday lives, and nurses need to understand how that might impact on older people and their care, and how to minimise or, preferably, erase ageism by challenging negative stereotypes.
- Increased numbers of older people, with more complex health- and social-care needs, require increased levels of skilled nursing care; however, finding such nurses in sufficient quantities is becoming increasingly challenging.
- Changes to our health- and social-care systems are needed in order to keep pace with the increasing numbers of older adults needing care.
- Nurses, wherever they work, must be able to provide evidence-based, person-centred care and evaluate its usefulness.
- Nurses need to grasp the opportunity to make positive change that will benefit older people and their families.

References

Abellan van Kan, G., Rolland, Y., Houles, M., Gillette-Guyonnet, S., Soto, M., and Vellas, B., 2010. The assessment of frailty in older adults. *Clinics in Geriatric Medicine*, 26 (2), 275-86.

Abhicharttibutra, K., Kunaviktikul, W., Turale, S., Wichaikhum, O.-A., and Srisuphan, W., 2017. Analysis of a government policy to address nursing shortage and nursing education quality. *International Nursing Review*, 64, 22-32.

Andrews, N., Gabbay, J., le May, A., Miller, E., O'Neill, M., and Petch, A., 2015. Developing evidence-enriched practice in health and social care with older people. JRF, York (April).

Bähler, C., Huber, C.A., Brüngger, B., and Reich, O., 2015. Multimorbidity, health care utilization and costs in an elderly community-dwelling population: a claims data based observational study. *BMC Health Services Research*, 15 (1), 23.

Barusch, A.S., 2013. The aging Tsunami: time for a new metaphor? *Journal of Gerontological Social Work*, 56 (3), 181-4.

Beard, J.R., Officer, A., De Carvalho, I.A., Sadana, R., Pot, A.M., Michel, J.P., Lloyd-Sherlock, P., Epping-Jordan, J.E., Peeters, G.M.E.E., Mahanani, W.R., Thiyagarajan, J.A., and Chatterji, S., 2016. The World report on ageing and health: a policy framework for healthy ageing. *The Lancet*, 387 (10033), 2145-54.

Blood, I., 2013. A better life: valuing our later years. JRF, York (December).

Blood, I., et al., 2010. Older people with high support needs: How can we empower them to enjoy a better life. JRF. Available at: www.jrf.org.uk/publications/better-life-high-support-needs

Boyd, C.M., Darer, J., Boult, C., Fried, L.P., Boult, L., and Wu, A.W., 2005. Clinical practice guidelines and quality of care for older patients with multiple comorbid diseases: implications for pay for performance. *JAMA*, 294 (6), 716-24.

Bridges, J., and Nugus, P., 2010. Dignity and significance in urgent care: older people's experiences. *Journal of Research in Nursing*, 15 (1), 43-53. doi: 10.1177/1744987109353522

Buchan, J., Duffield, C., and Jordan, A., 2015. 'Solving' nursing shortages: do we need a new agenda? *Journal of Nursing Management*, 23 (5), 543-5.

Butler, R.N., 1969. Age-ism: another form of bigotry. *The Gerontologist*, 9 (4), 243-6.

Butler, R.N., 2002. *Why survive? Being old in America*. Baltimore: Johns Hopkins University Press.

Calnan, M., Tadd, W., Calnan, A., Hilllman, A., Read, S., and Bayer, A., 2013. 'I often worry about the older person being in that system': exploring the key influences on the provision of dignified care for older people in acute hospitals. *Ageing and Society*, 33 (3), 465-85.

Canada, 2017. Registered Nurses Profile (including Nurse Practitioners), Canada, 2017. Available at: www.cna-aiic.ca/en/nursing-practice/the-practice-of-nursing/health-human-resources/nursing-statistics/canada [Accessed 13 May 2019].

Canadian Institute for Health Information (CIHI), 2010. Health care in Canada 2010. Canadian Institute for Health Information (CIHI), Ontario.

Canadian Institute for Health Information (CIHI), 2011. Health care in Canada, 2011: a focus on seniors and aging. Canadian Institute for Health Information (CIHI), Ontario.

Canadian Institute for Health Information (CIHI), 2016. Measuring patient harm in Canadian hospitals. Canadian Institute for Health Information (CIHI), Ontario.

Charise, A., 2012. Old age and the crisis of capacity. *Occasion: Interdisciplinary Studies in the Humanities, 4*, 1-16.

Conference Board of Canada, 2013. Future care for Canadian seniors—why it matters. The Conference Board of Canada, October, 1-10.

de la Rue, M.B., 2003. Preventing ageism in nursing students: an action theory approach. *Australian Journal of Advanced Nursing*, 20, 8-14.

Dewar, B., and Kennedy, C., 2016. Strategies for enhancing "Person Knowledge" in an older people care setting. *Western Journal of Nursing Research*, 38 (11), 1469-88.

Dewar, B., and Nolan, M., 2013. Caring about caring: developing a model to implement compassionate relationship centred care in an older people care setting. *International Journal of Nursing Studies*, 50 (9), 1247-58.

Elbourne, H.F., Hominick, K., Mallery, L., and Rockwood, K., 2013. Characteristics of patients described as sub-acute in an Acute Care Hospital. *Canadian Journal on Aging / La Revue canadienne du vieillissement*, 32 (2), 203-8.

Ferrario, C.G., Freeman, F.J., Nellett, G., and Scheel, J., 2007. Changing nursing students' attitudes about aging: an argument for the successful aging paradigm. *Educational Gerontology*, 34 (1), 51-66.

Fillmore Elbourne, H., and le May, A., 2015. Crafting intermediate care: one team's journey towards integration and innovation. *Journal of Research in Nursing*, 20 (1), 56-71.

Gould, O.N., Dupuis-Blanchard, S., and MacLennan, A., 2015. Canadian nursing students and the care of older patients. *Journal of Applied Gerontology*, 34 (6), 797-814.

Gould, O.N., MacLennan, A., and Dupuis-Blanchard, S., 2012. Career preferences of nursing students. *Canadian Journal on Aging / La Revue canadienne du vieillissement*, 31 (4), 471-82.

Haight, B.K., Christ, M.A., and Dias, J.K., 1994. Does nursing education promote ageism? *Journal of Advanced Nursing*, 20 (2), 382-90.

Herdman, E., 2002. Challenging the discourses of nursing ageism. *International Journal of Nursing Studies*, 39 (1), 105-14.

Hirst, S.P., and Lane, A.M., 2016. How do nursing students perceive the needs of older clients? Addressing a knowledge gap. *Journal of Geriatrics*, 2016, Article ID 7546753, 7 pages. https://doi.org/10.1155/2016/7546753.

Hoffman, C., Rice, D., and Sung, H.Y., 1996. Persons with chronic conditions. Their prevalence and costs. *JAMA*, 276 (18), 1473–9.

Hominick, K., McLeod, V., and Rockwood, K., 2016. Characteristics of older adults admitted to hospital versus those discharged home, in emergency department patients referred to internal medicine. *Canadian Geriatrics Journal*, 19 (1), 9–14.

Humphries, R., 2015. Integrated health and social care in England – progress and prospects. *Health Policy*, 119 (7), 856–59.

Humphries, N., Brugha, R., and McGee, H., 2012. Nurse migration and health workforce planning: Ireland as illustrative of international challenges. *Health Policy*, 107 (1), 44–53.

Katz, J., Holland, C., Peace, S., and Taylor, E., 2011. *A better life: what older people with high support needs value*. Joseph Rowntree Foundation, York.

Kingma, M., 2007. Nurses on the move: A global overview. *Health Services Research*, 42, 1281–98. doi:10.1111/j.1475-6773.2007.00711.x.

Krichbaum, K., Kaas, M.J., Wyman, J.F., and Van Son, C.R., 2015. Facilitated learning to advance geriatrics: increasing the capacity of nurse faculty to teach students about caring for older adults. *The Gerontologist*, 55 (Suppl 1), S154–64.

Marengoni, A., Angleman, S., Melis, R., Mangialasche, F., Karp, A., and Garmen, A., 2011. Aging with multimorbidity: a systematic review of the literature. *Ageing Research Reviews*, 10 (4), 430–9.

Martin, R., Williams, C., and O'Neill, D., 2009. Retrospective analysis of attitudes to ageing in the Economist: apocalyptic demography for opinion formers. *BMJ* (Clinical research ed.), 339, b4914.

Melillo, K.D., 2017. Geropsychiatric nursing: what's in your toolkit? *Journal of Gerontological Nursing*, 43 (1), 3–6.

Mezey, M., Capezuti, E., and Fulmer, T., 2004. Care of older adults. *Nursing Clinics of North America*, 39 (3), xiii–xx.

Nuernberger, K., Atkinson, S., and MacDonald, G., 2018. Seniors in transition: exploring pathways across the care continuum. *Healthcare Quarterly*, 21 (1), 10–12.

Nunnelee, J., Tanner, E.I., Cotton, A., Harris, M., Alderman, J., Hassler, L., Conley, D., and Schumacher, S., 2015. NGNA: position paper on essential gerontological nursing education in registered nursing and continuing education programs. *Geriatric Nursing*, 36 (3), 239–41.

O'Brien-Pallas, L., Murphy, G.T., Shamian, J., Li, X., and Hayes, L.J., 2010. Impact and determinants of nurse turnover: a pan-Canadian study. *Journal of Nursing Management*, 18 (8), 1073–86.

Officer, A., Schneiders, M.L., Wu, D., Nash, P., Thiyagarajan, J.A., and Beard, J.R., 2016. Valuing older people: time for a global campaign to combat ageism. *Bulletin of the World Health Organization*, 94 (10), 710–10A.

Oostrom, S.H., Picavet, H.S., Bruin, S.R., Stirbu, I., Korevaar, J.C., and Schellevis, F.G., 2014. Multimorbidity of chronic diseases and health care utilization in general practice. *BMC Family Practice*, 15, 61.

Oliver, D., 2018. Ghost wards and rota gaps show the need for official safe staffing levels. *BMJ*, 361 (May), k2322.

Paez, K.A., Zhao, L., and Hwang, W., 2009. Rising out-of-pocket spending for chronic conditions: a ten-year trend. *Health Affairs* (Millwood), 28 (1), 15–25.

Prentice, D., Boscart, V., McGilton, K.S., and Escrig, A., 2017. Factors influencing new RNs' supervisory performance in long-term care facilities. *Canadian Journal on Aging / La Revue canadienne du vieillissement*, 36 (4), 463–71.

Prohaska, T., Belansky, E., Belza, B., Buchner, D., Marshall, V., McTigue, K., Satariano, W., and Wilcox, S., 2006. Physical activity, public health, and aging: critical issues and research priorities. *The Journals of Gerontology: Series B*, 61 (5), S267–73.

RCN, 2017. The UK nursing labour market review 2017. Royal College of Nursing, London, 28.

Rechel, B., Doyle, Y., Grundy, E., and Mckee, M., 2009. How can health systems respond to population ageing? Policy Brief 10. WHO Europe.

Rockwood, K., and Mitnitski, A., 2011. Frailty defined by deficit accumulation and geriatric medicine defined by frailty. *Clinics in Geriatric Medicine*, 27 (1), 17–26.

Rockwood, K., Song, X., MacKnight, C., Bergman, H., Hogan, D.B., McDowell, I., and Mitnitski, A., 2005. A global clinical measure of fitness and frailty in elderly people. *CMAJ : Canadian Medical Association Journal / journal de l'Association medicale canadienne*, 173 (5), 489–95.

Steis, M.R., Shaughnessy, M., and Gordon, S.M., 2012. Delirium: a very common problem you may not recognize. *Journal of Psychosocial Nursing and Mental Health Services*, 50 (7), 17–20.

WHO, 2009a. World population ageing. United Nations Department of Economic & Social Affairs Population Division.

WHO, 2009b. Global health risks: mortality and burden of disease attributable to selected major risks. Bulletin of the World Health Organization.

WHO, 2011. Global health and ageing. U.S. National Institute of Aging.

WHO, 2013a. Global action plan for the prevention and control of noncommunicable diseases 2013–2020. World Health Organization.

WHO, 2013b. The world health report 2013: research for universal health coverage. World Health Organization Press. ISBN: 978 92 4 156459 5

WHO, 2015a. WHO World report on ageing and health 2015. World Health Organization.

WHO, 2015b. World health statistic. Current opinion in genetics and development.

WHO, 2015c. WHO noncommunicable diseases [online]. Fact sheet. http://origin.who.int/mediacentre/factsheets/fs355/en/

WHO, 2017. Global strategy and action plan on ageing and health. www.who.int/ageing/global-strategy/en/.

Wolff, J.L., Starfield, B., and Anderson, G., 2002. Prevalence, expenditures, and complications of multiple chronic conditions in the elderly. *Archives of Internal Medicine*, 162 (20), 2269–76.

World Health Assembly 64, 2011. Strengthening nursing and midwifery. World Health Organization.

Worsfold, B., Prohaska T.R., Anderson L.A., and Binstock R.H., editors., 2013. *Public health for an aging society*. Baltimore, MD: John Hopkins University Press. *Canadian Journal on Aging / La Revue canadienne du vieillissement*, 32 (2), 221-222.

3 Stories of older age

Andrée le May and Heather Fillmore Elbourne

Introduction

For some people old age is signalled by retirement from paid work, or having grandchildren, or feeling less active, or getting to a 'special' age and celebrating with a party, or feeling rejuvenated by opportunities that weren't available before—more leisure time, more energy, more freedom, or courage to do what one had always wanted to (www.theguardian.com/society/2018/nov/17/age-nothing-do-with-it-transition-later-life-transgender). Old age, *per se*, is not necessarily a gloomy time despite sometimes being portrayed as such in the media. However, for some older people, as they get frailer physically, socially, and/or mentally they begin to feel less resilient and sometimes more melancholy. Being old is an individual experience, and we believe that knowing more about older people's experiences will help nurses to be more sensitive to each person's needs, as well as understand better some of the cross-cutting problems and difficulties that older people and their families/carers face. Some clinicians call these challenges the 'geriatric giants' e.g. immobility, instability, incontinence, and impaired intellect/memory—they focus largely on impairment and its correction (or not), and whilst the impact of these cannot be ignored for many older people[1] we wanted to start with a different set of experiences to show the power of positive care and the impact that person-centred, respectful care has on the people involved in it. To do this we have selected some stories of older people, or as the person who compiled these stories, Nick Andrews, calls them "magic moments".

The magic moments we have chosen set a backdrop for the clinical stories in the remainder of the book. They show positive aspects of older people's care experiences and emphasise how meaningful and special experiences can come from seemingly simple and "small" aspects of care. They are presented without commentary to ensure that it is each reader's interpretation/meaning rather than ours that remains with them as they read on. You will all have your own stories to remember and tell as long as you allow yourself time to listen.

Some "magic moments" focused on older people with dementia (Andrews 2018a)

A dementia or designer label?

A woman who lives with advanced dementia moved into our care home. She has limited communication and comprehension. When getting to know about her past life, we were told that she originally came from Austria and then moved to London in the 1970s to work as a seamstress for the fashion guru Dame Vivienne Westwood.

Finding out about this woman's rich life history has given us a window to connect with her, and whenever we mention Vivienne Westwood's name her face lights up. She may not be able to find the words, but she clearly experiences the positive feelings that this name and associated memories bring.

We are now researching Vivienne Westwood fashion from the 1970s and developing this lady's own life story scrap book. By connecting through life-story work, we have been able to see the woman behind the label of 'dementia'. She now has a 'fashion designer' label. As a result we can now enrich her life and celebrate her wonderful memories.

Are you my sister?

On a shopping trip to a local supermarket, a retired nurse who lives with advanced dementia pushed her trolley around, filling it up with cheese, milk, a plant, and biscuits. When we got back to the bus she sat down next to me, looked at me and asked, "Are you my sister?", to which I replied "Something like that". She smiled, linked her arm through mine and gestured to me to open-up my purse. She then took 50 pence and gave it to the driver, saying "Go buy yourself an ice-cream". Never undermine the importance of feeling safe in relationships, and having a sense of significance and belonging.

Little, unexpected things

I got chatting to a 97-year-old woman living with dementia about the things she grew in her garden. She told me that she used to make green tomato chutney. I asked her if she would like me to get her some, to which she replied "Oh yes please!" Her whole face lit up. After much searching I managed to get hold of a jar. When I handed it to her, a tear rolled down her face, but also a big smile appeared. She decided that she would like a cheese and green tomato chutney sandwich for tea. This woman was able to reconnect with her memories and share them with me. Remembering what mattered to her enabled her to experience one of her favourite things which she hadn't been able to for many years and created a connection between us.

Until death us do part

A man in our service who lived with dementia asked me for a pencil and tape measure which he could see on the desk. I did not know why he wanted them, but gave them to him. From that day on he did not put them down. For a start, he used them to measure the floor with a big smile on his face as he did so. When his wife came to visit she commented that she had seen a big improvement in his mood, as he was constantly smiling and busy, measuring and recording information. This man then began to measure the staff as well. When we mentioned this to his wife, she told us that before he retired he had been an undertaker and that he was probably measuring us up for our coffins! This man had been an undertaker since he was 14 and this had been the family business for many genera-tions. A small plastic tape measure and pencil had made all the difference to this man, through which we were able to support him in achieving a sense of familiarity, purpose and achievement.

Some "magic moments" focused on depression and loneliness (Andrews 2018b)

Can we cwtch?

I met a man in his home who was very depressed. Although he had previously been able to manage his health, finance and personal care, he had given up. He was obviously experiencing severe depression, and began to sob, telling me that he didn't want to be here anymore. I did my best to comfort and re-assure him, and was touched by his deep heartache. The man was completely shrouded by his duvet as he expressed his deeply sad emotions. He asked me for a cwtch*, which I gladly gave, and he continued to sob as I comforted him. However, after a while he became more composed and was able to summon up strength to make the decision to accept our help and come into our service.

Over time, day by day and little by little, he has begun to settle into our service and has started to develop trust and confidence. Although this man initially would not come out of his room, he is now starting to do more for himself and has begun to build trusting relationships. He is now accessing community facilities and going out shopping supported by staff. We have started to notice him gradually rebuilding his skills which he had lost through his depression. It is heart-warming and very rewarding to us all to see this man's confidence grow as we watch him progress to independent living.

*cwtch is a Welsh word for hug.

The power of a pop-in

An older woman, living on her own had become isolated from family and friends. She was introduced to a weekly group called 'Roll and Stroll', which is held at the Café on Swansea Bay with a fantastic sea view. She attended the group regularly and was able to meet new people while also having fun exercising.

However, as good as this all is, her personal 'Magic Moment' came after a recent period of ill health, during which time she could not attend the group. She told me how she had been overwhelmed, because members of the group had taken time to ring her or pop-in to check how she was. "Nobody has ever really cared about me before. It meant so much to me, and encouraged me to get better and get back to my Roll and Stroll group of friends.

Note

1 There are many stories of older people's health experience on the healthtalk-on-line website (www.healthtalk.org/peoples-experiences), and we have collected some in Appendix 1.

References

Andrews N (2018a) Magic Moments in Care Homes.
Andrews N (2018b) Magic Moments in Adult Service Provision.
Both booklets are available from Nick Andrews at N.D.Andrews@swansea.ac.uk

4 Risk taking and risk aversion

Imogen Blood

Introduction

The importance of assessing and managing 'risks' has moved up the agenda in recent years, both in health care and in other areas of our lives. For health professionals, this can be accompanied by a fear of getting it wrong, resulting in injury or death, and the investigations, litigation, and disciplinary action that may follow. Given this, there can be a tendency to err on the side of caution, to play it safe, to be risk averse.

However, decisions which may appear to be 'risk averse' can also have harmful consequences: admitting someone to hospital 'to be on the safe side' may increase their risk of catching an infection, or in the case of an older person with dementia, of them becoming disorientated and having a fall whilst on the ward. Older people who have ended up staying in hospital for a long time run the risk of losing their muscle tone and confidence to walk. Although moving to a care home may seem to be a 'safer' option for an older person who has become frail or developed memory problems, this overlooks the emotional and social impact of leaving their home, their belongings, their neighbours, and their independence. Encouraging someone to sit on a commode rather than get up and walk to the toilet may reduce the risk of falling, but it incurs a number of what Clarke and her colleagues (2011) have termed 'hidden harms'.

In recent qualitative research conducted with older people living in the community and in care homes (Blood & Litherland 2015; Blood et al. 2016), older people focus on:

- The risk of losing your independence, having to leave your home, becoming highly dependent on other people, or becoming a 'burden' to your family;
- The risk of social isolation, often caused by disability, depression, poverty, fear of crime, bereavement, discrimination and difference, and lack of transport and rurality;
- The risk of not being able to do the things that 'make you tick'–from keeping your house and garden in order, and continuing to play a role in your community or family, to hobbies and simple pleasures; and
- The risk of 'losing your confidence'.

Nursing older people can throw up a number of dilemmas in which we must be accountable for 'managing' different types of risks, while remaining focused on the central importance of respecting older people's rights to autonomy, dignity, and equality. Sometimes this means having to swim upstream in a culture which sees older people as 'vulnerable' and our role as 'protecting' them.

In this chapter, we explore various dilemmas relating to risk, using stories to explore the legal context and the principles which both the law and good practice suggest. We present and apply a number of different practice 'tools', which can support you to have more balanced conversations about risk with families and colleagues, to enable older people to do the things that matter to them, and to help you to think about the emotional impact of working with complexity, where there often is not one clear 'right' answer.

Supporting people to do the things that really matter to them: Pat's story

Pat is 91 years old and has been living in a nursing home for the past year. She has Chronic Obstructive Pulmonary Disease, for which she is required to take regular oxygen, and, given her limited vision and mobility, it was no longer viable for her to continue living alone. Despite her health challenges, Pat has always had a positive outlook and she is cheery and popular. She loves music, and she and her late husband used to sing together in clubs and bars.

One of Pat's sons dies suddenly of a heart attack and Pat is devastated. Her grandsons are organising a music night to celebrate his life and raise money for a heart research charity. When Pat receives an invite, her eyes light up for the first time in months. Graham—one of the nurses who is closest to Pat—is determined that he will do everything possible to support Pat to go to the music night, even though it is over an hour's drive away. However, when he goes to discuss it with the care home manager, she is not convinced—the risks are too high and it will require at least two staff members to accompany her: the home cannot spare that many staff for a whole evening.

Graham is not deterred—he says that he doesn't mind giving up his own evening to go along with Pat to the event, but—although he jokes with Pat about 'sneaking her down the fire escape'—he realises that he will need his manager's blessing to take Pat and her oxygen tank out of the building. He remembers a training session he attended a while ago with the council on and digs out his notes.... 'Positive Risk Taking' is defined as:

> Weighing up the potential benefits and harms of exercising one choice of action over another. Identifying the potential risks involved (i.e. good risk assessment) and developing plans and actions (i.e. good risk management) that reflect the positive potentials and stated priorities of the service user (i.e. a strengths approach). It involves using "available" resources and support to achieve the desired outcomes, and to minimise the potential harmful outcomes.
>
> (Morgan & Andrews 2016, p. 128)

Key principles of positive risk taking

- Decision-making about risk should be balanced; in other words, we should look at the benefits of taking a risk (and the potential harms of not taking it) as well as the harms which might occur if something goes wrong, being specific about what these are.

- We should aim to make and record decisions which are defensible (i.e. well-founded and justifiable) not defensive (i.e. which we can use to protect ourselves and our agencies).
- We should work collaboratively with older people, their families, and across agencies to make decisions about risk, using all available resources.

Graham makes some phone calls and invites a few key people to a meeting to discuss this; in addition to himself and Pat, he persuades his manager to come, along with Pat's general practitioner (GP), her grandson and his partner, and a couple of carers from the home. He comes up with a list of questions, based on his course materials, to structure the meeting. The manager chairs the meeting and goes around the room, giving each person a chance to say what they think about each question. Graham takes notes.

Key questions

1   **Our hopes**: What are the potential benefits of Pat going to the music night?
2   **Our fears**: What could go wrong? How likely is this to happen, and how severe might the impact be if it did?
3   **Risk management**: What would need to happen to reduce these risks to a point where everyone feels sufficiently reassured?
4   **Resources**: What resources do we have—both within services, but also within the family and the community/voluntary sector—to make the trip possible and to manage the risks?
5   **Contingency planning**: What will we do if we encounter problems?
6   **Review**: Under what circumstances should we review this plan?

A few points and observations

- Sharing risks and making decisions collectively in this way can help to reduce fears and come up with ideas and resources that we might not otherwise have considered. This could be about bringing together a group of relevant professionals and non-professionals to discuss a particular individual or decision, as in Pat's case. It might also be about creating a 'Community of Practice' to support positive risk taking.

A 'Community of Practice' is a group of people who share a particular concern or passion and interact with each other, through meetings and/or social media to learn from and support each other in changing the way things are done.

- In some settings, staff end up doing things 'under the radar' and outside of work in order to support older people to take positive risks, because it would go against their organisation's policies. Although this is well-intentioned, it can then create other risks, especially if things do not go as planned.

Recognising that professional boundaries policies were creating a barrier to connecting with older people and supporting them to do the things that mattered to them, health- and social-care professionals in South Wales worked with groups of older people and family carers to review and change their policies (Andrews et al. 2015). For further resources and stories about this project, see http://deep-resources.chrismog.co.uk/#Stories_and_Quotes.

Motivating a patient to be less risk averse: Cassie's story

Cassie is 82 and lives alone. She was discharged from hospital a couple of weeks ago, following surgery on a fall-induced hip fracture. Maryam is a district nurse who has been asked to assess and treat Cassie for pressure sores. According to her notes, at the point of discharge from hospital, Cassie was able to stand up independently using a walking frame and take a couple of steps. She has been receiving three visits a day from carers to assist with personal care and eating, and has been seen once by a physiotherapist since returning home.

Maryam goes out to visit Cassie, examines the sores, and dresses them. She asks Cassie how often she is moving from her chair during the day. Cassie explains that she daren't move by herself unless the carers are present because she is terrified she will fall again, so she is sitting in the chair for long periods of time. Sometimes she manages to transfer herself onto the commode which carers leave next to the chair; but she is also using incontinence pads. Cassie's mood seems very low, and she seems to be smoking heavily.

Maryam asks what the physiotherapist has told her to do—he has given her some chair-based exercises and suggested that she practises standing up and taking a step or two using her walking frame as often as she can—at least six times a day. Cassie explains that she started off doing the chair-based exercises, but they were painful and she did not see the point of them. The carers are supposed to help her stand up and move around, but this takes quite a long time and they have a lot of other tasks to do during their short visits.

Maryam points out that, although she can understand why Cassie is anxious about falling, sitting in her chair like this is not risk-free. In the short term, these sores are being caused because she is staying in one place for too long. In the longer term, it is really important for Cassie to build the muscle up around the hip joint and throughout her body if her hip is to heal properly and she is to regain her mobility and independence. At this, Cassie becomes very upset—she says that she blames herself for falling in the first place because she was 'being stupid' trying to reach something down off a shelf; now she feels she has 'blown it'—she will never get her old life back.

What might Maryam do to help Cassie 'get her old life back'?

Messages from research

For the majority of older people, maintaining independence is a key motivator influencing actions (Gardiner et al. 2017).

Cassie may feel that she has lost all independence now and there is no prospect of regaining it. In order to become motivated again, she needs to believe and see that recovery and progress is possible.

Horton (2007) interviewed older people (women, in particular) who chastised and blamed themselves for falling. Carefulness was seen as a 'protective strategy' for them, in which the individual exerts 'personal control' by restricting their activity and being very cautious not to take further risks.

This suggests that Maryam's focus should be on helping Cassie to *take back control* in a way that does not attempt to close down all risk of falling.

McMillan et al. (2014) interviewed 19 older people returning home from hospital following a fall-induced hip fracture and explored the different ways in which they 'balanced risks' in order to 'take control'. Most of the people they interviewed, like Cassie:

> passed through a period of heightened foreboding, especially when they returned home and were reminded of the location of the fall. They perceived their environment to be precarious, having to balance risk for themselves instead of relying on healthcare professionals. As a consequence, they raised the level of their protective guarding.
>
> (p. 252)

Some of this group decided that the 'orders' they had been given (in Cassie's case, by the physiotherapist) were too risky—they 'took control' and disregarded them (McMillan et al. 2014, p. 253).

McMillan et al. found that people were best supported to balance risks appropriately when they received good information, advice, feedback, and reassurance about their progress from health professionals—in a way that was positive, constructive, and gave control back.

Introduction to motivational interviewing

'Motivational Interviewing' is a set of skills for supporting people to build on their own motivation to make changes in their lives. It can be particularly helpful where someone feels ambivalent or torn between a number of options. It involves guiding people and helping them reflect on what matters to them and what they are concerned about, without telling them what to do. It's not about 'tricking' people into making changes; rather it recognises that each person is an expert in their situation and ultimately needs to make and be responsible for their own choices (Blood & Guthrie 2018).

Motivational interviewing involves:

- Actively listening and reflecting back content, meaning and feelings;
- Asking open-ended questions to understand what motivates the person and what concerns they have;
- Affirming the things that matter to the person, their strengths, and skills; and
- Summarising what you have heard, especially where there is ambivalence.

Further reading: The Royal College of Nursing's website contains a number of resources on 'Motivational Interviewing', as part of their Supporting Behaviour Change programme (www.rcn.org.uk/clinical-topics/supporting-behaviour-change).

A sample motivational interviewing conversation with Cassie

Maryam:	(open question) What is it about your 'old life' that you are particularly keen to get back?
Cassie:	Well—all of it really! Look at me sitting here, I can't do anything for myself, I can't go anywhere, the only people I ever see are the paid carers.
Maryam:	(reflection) So, it's important to you to be independent, and be able to get out and see other people?
Cassie:	Yes, I've always been a really independent person.
Maryam:	(affirmation) Your independence really matters to you.
Cassie:	Yes, it always has. Losing it is the hardest part of getting older.
Maryam:	(reflection) So, you'd really like to work on regaining your independence and be able to be get out and do things for yourself again.
Cassie:	Well, I obviously need to be able to walk again!
Maryam:	(open question) What's your understanding of what needs to happen for you to be able to walk again?
Cassie:	A miracle!? Well this hip needs to heal up and I need to get my strength back, and my confidence I suppose. I don't even know whether that's possible....
Maryam:	(reflection) You feel as though you don't have enough information about recovery.
Cassie:	There was a lot going on in the hospital, I can't really remember what they told me and what they didn't.
Maryam:	(reflection) So, because there was a lot going on at the hospital, you can't really remember what the medical staff said to you about your recovery.
Cassie:	Yes, though the physio was clear that I need to do these exercises if I am to stand a chance of getting better.
Maryam:	(open question) OK, and how do you feel about doing the exercises?
Cassie:	They hurt and I don't know if they should hurt that much, so I worry about whether I am doing them right and whether I might be making things worse. And like I said, I am worried that if I start trying to stand up and walk when I am on my own, I might fall and then I would be back to square one.... Or maybe even worse.
Maryam:	(affirmation) It's hard for you to do something that hurts and scares you, when you are not even convinced it is doing you good, and might risk making it worse.
Cassie:	Yes. But I feel like I have given up too easily and that is making me feel sad.
Maryam:	(reflection) You feel sad that you haven't been able to do the exercises.
Cassie:	Yes.... and cross with myself.
Maryam:	(open question) What do you think needs to happen for you to start doing the exercises and keep doing them?
Cassie:	I guess it would be easier if there was someone there to encourage me and tell me if I am doing them right—just for a few times, at least. And I need to get my determined head on.... Perhaps I need to understand that there is hope that I can get better.

Maryam:	(reflection) So you need to feel that there is hope.
Cassie:	I suppose knowing that there are other people who have been through this and managed to get back on their feet.
Maryam:	(summary) So, just to check I've understood, your independence really matters to you. You'd like to be able to do the exercises, so that you can strengthen your hip, but you feel that you need some more support and encouragement. You'd like to know whether other people have been able to recover from similar injuries, so that you can feel more hopeful.
Cassie:	Yes, that's right
Maryam:	(open question) So, what sorts of things will you ask the physiotherapist at your next appointment?
Cassie:	Whether I am doing the exercises right, what is causing this pain, how quickly I might expect to see some progress if I can make myself do them, and whether he thinks I will be able to walk again.
Maryam:	(affirmation) It will be really motivating for you if the physiotherapist is able to tell you about some of the other people he has worked with, and how their recovery has gone.
Cassie:	Yes, I think that would help. I think I might see if my daughter can come with me to that appointment. She lives about an hour away and can only really get over occasionally, but maybe if she could come and help me remember what he says and how to do the exercises, she can help me do them a few times when we get back.
Maryam:	Well that sounds like a good plan. So, I will come back on Tuesday and find out how you have got on with all of that. And in the meantime, I would like to make a referral to an occupational therapist—they will come and look around your house with you and see if there are any changes that could be made to help reduce your chances of falling in the future.

Mind your language!

Some of the language used to talk about or with older people implies a judgement about risk. For example,

- When we describe a person living with dementia as 'wandering', we imply that their walking is pointless, and therefore a risk not worth taking.
- When we describe the behaviour of a person with dementia as 'disturbing' or 'challenging', we are focusing on the impact it has on *us*, rather than what the person might be trying to express.
- 'Old dears' and 'little old' people suggest a need to be protected.
- '*Still* driving' and '*still* doing your own gardening' imply that a person would normally be expected to have stopped these activities by this age.
- Labelling someone as 'a faller' or describing them as being 'vulnerable' or 'at risk' suggests that risks are somehow unavoidably contained within them, rather than specific to particular situations they might be in. Any of us can be 'vulnerable' in some situations, very few people are 'vulnerable' in all situations.

Becoming more aware of the impact of the language we use and gently challenging others to do the same is not 'political correctness gone mad'; it is a first step to having more balanced conversations about risk with older people, their families, and other professionals.

Derek's story

Derek was diagnosed with Alzheimer's disease several years ago and lives with his wife Bernie. Recently, he has started—in the words of his wife—to go 'wandering'. Last night, the Police eventually found him, after four hours' searching. They brought him to A&E since they were concerned that he might be hypothermic and he had some surface wounds which needed dressing. He has been admitted to a ward, where Rohina is the Senior Nurse in charge.

Derek's son, Jim, and daughter, Eleanor, come in to visit him on the ward and ask to see Rohina to find out about his condition. Rohina reassures them that his condition is stable and that he is just being kept in for monitoring—with any luck, he will be fit for discharge within a day or two. Jim is horrified at the prospect of his father going back to live at home and believes that his Dad should now be placed in a more secure setting: the risks of this happening again are just too high. Eleanor is unsure—she knows how much her parents would hate to be separated from each other, though she can also see how exhausted and stressed her mother is. Rohina phones the hospital social-work team to discuss the case.

What are the key questions and considerations here?

1   What is the purpose and meaning to Derek of walking?

When Vallelly and her colleagues (2006) interviewed care staff in extra care housing schemes they described how tenants living with dementia would 'wander' and risk getting lost as a result. However, when Vallelly interviewed tenants with dementia, they explained that they were walking with purpose—for exercise and to get out of their flats and meet other people.

As June Andrews (2017) argues:

> Our problem is that we don't know what the purpose is, so it appears to be pointless, unless you understand what the person is thinking. Even if you discover that their purpose is futile, such as setting off for work, decades after retirement, or trying to visit long-dead friends, there is a lot that can be done to help.
>
> (p. 322)

Andrews advises us to consider:

- Where the person says they are going, if asked at the time?
- The pace and intensity with which they set out: do they appear calm, purposeful, confused, or agitated?
- Whether there seem to be particular triggers (e.g. Bernie being out of sight) or times of day?
- Whether the walks seem part of a general sense of restlessness, e.g. in which the person paces and moves around a lot?

Starting to reflect on Derek's behaviour in this way can shift the whole focus of the discussion from an assumption that the 'wandering' is an inherently harmful activity to something which has a function for Derek. If we can try to understand the function, it should become clearer whether the focus should be on facilitating him to go for these walks, but in a safer way, or finding ways of reducing the stress which is prompting him to get out and move.

'Facilitating walks in a safer way' might include:

- Someone going with him, perhaps for planned walks.
- Exploring how technology might be used in a way that everyone, including Derek, agrees with. Simple solutions might include: a mobile phone or other device with GPS tracking, or a wristband with embedded contact information, which someone who finds him could retrieve using their phone, e.g. a 'Dementia Buddy', http://dementiabuddy.co.uk/guardian-angel.php.

Reducing stress might include:

- Making sure Derek is busy and occupied with something he enjoys doing.
- Regular reassurance and 'anchoring'—for example, a simple technological solution could be set up so that, every time the front door is opened, a recording of Bernie's voice says, "Derek, I'm in the house—don't go out without telling me!"
- Use of personalised sounds, smells, images, etc., which calm Derek—this might include Bernie putting on his favourite music or TV programme whenever she needs to leave the room for a period of time.

2   Should Derek return home or go into a care home?

First, it is important to be absolutely clear about whose decision this is to make—this will differ under different legal circumstances; however, unless Derek has been sectioned, it will always be crucial to try to ascertain what *he* wants, or what he would have wanted if he is deemed to lack capacity and a 'best interests' decision is being considered to deprive him of his liberty (SCIE 2017).

In the following section, the key legal powers, duties, and responsibilities in the English and Welsh contexts are summarised. Readers from other countries should check the equivalent legislation; however, the good practice principles should be transferable.

Rights, responsibilities, duties, and powers

Mental Health Act (England and Wales)

A person with dementia can be sectioned to remain in hospital under the Mental Health Act, on the authorisation of an Approved Mental Health Professional and two doctors to allow for full assessment (under Section 2) or to receive treatment (under Section 3) (Alzheimer's Society 2018).

Mental Capacity Act (England and Wales)

Under the Mental Capacity Act (MCA), a person's capacity to make decisions should be assessed. Mental capacity—especially in people with dementia—tends to fluctuate, and different decisions will have greater implications than others. The more serious the decision, the more formal the assessment of capacity needs to be (usually involving a GP, a consultant psychologist/psychiatrist, and/or a specialist social worker).

The MCA says that a person is unable to make their own decision if they cannot do one or more of the following four things:

- Understand information given to them.
- Retain that information long enough to be able to make the decision.
- Weigh up the information available to make the decision.
- Communicate their decision—this could be by talking and using sign language or even simple muscle movements such as blinking an eye or squeezing a hand.

Key principles of the MCA are:

- You should start from the assumption that the person **does** have the capacity to make the decision in question.
- Just because they are making what you believe is an unwise decision, it does not necessarily follow that they lack the capacity to make it.
- All efforts should be made to find ways of communicating with someone, both to give them the information they need to make a decision and to communicate their wishes.
- Remember that capacity or lack of it is decision-specific: a person does not permanently 'lack capacity' (assuming they are conscious).

Where someone is assessed as lacking the capacity to make a decision, you should check whether they have made a lasting power of attorney, which gives—usually a family member—the right to make decisions on their behalf.

If not, then a 'best interests' decision should be made on their behalf by a suitably trained professional, drawing on the knowledge of family and friends. If there are no friends and family, or there are very different views amongst them, an Independent Mental Capacity Advocate (IMCA) should be appointed.

If a person (who has not been sectioned under the Mental Health Act) is being constantly supervised and controlled and is not free to leave either a hospital or a care home, authorisation must be sought from the local authority for a deprivation of liberty.

Duty of care in relation to hospital discharge

The Parliamentary and Health Service Ombudsman (2016) sets out a number of principles in relation to effective hospital discharge, based on learning from their most serious investigations in England. These include:

- Start discharge/transfer planning as soon after admission as possible.
- Involve patients and family carers: make sure they have the right information to inform decision-making and hear their concerns about whether they feel they will be able to cope at home.
- Work effectively in partnership with Adult Social Care, especially where a person might lack the mental capacity to make a decision or where there are concerns about their ability to cope at home after discharge.

- Inform carers (family members, housing/care staff) when a person is due to be discharged.
- Arrange follow-up by community health services.

Tips for supporting decision-making about risk

Different family members and professionals can have different views in cases like Derek's, and sometimes these change over time. It is not Rohina's role to make the decision, but she will clearly have influence here, and can use this to challenge and support family members and other professionals.

- Sometimes it can be helpful to **stop talking about 'risks' and start talking about 'worries' or 'fears' and 'hopes'**. What are we worried about? How worried are we? What can we do to reduce these worries?
- As Robinson et al. (2007) point out, 'the discourse that underpins health policy and guidance views risk as something real and objective that can be measured and acted upon' (p. 390). Similarly, Finlayson (2015) argues, 'The very paradigm of risk drives expectations of management and intervention. Talk of human worries drives relationships and discussion' (p. 1).
- Look at the potential for benefits and harms from each course of action: it is easy to focus only on the risks of going back home, but what about the risks of going into a care home? We know that, especially for a person with dementia, such a move—even into a really well-run home—can be extremely disorientating.
- Don't focus only on the possible physical harms which might arise from a course of action and overlook the likelihood of emotional, psychological, and social harm. Derek might be physically safer in a locked wing of a care home, but what might the impact be on his mental well-being, his relationship with Bernie, and his quality of life?

   The following very simple tool could be used to capture the hopes and fears of each member of the family/multi-agency team:

Individuals	Fears and hopes	Returning home	Going into a care home
Derek	Fears		
	Hopes		
Bernie *Add more rows for others*	Fears		
	Hopes		

Source: Adapted from Blood and Guthrie (2018).

- Think about who else might be involved in supporting Derek and Bernie on discharge: this could include:
   o The Police (who might want to take a photo and some details of Derek and advise Bernie to notify them sooner if he goes missing again).
   o Local dementia charities, such as the Alzheimer's Society and/or carers' groups, who could offer advice and support to the family on what is available in their area—this might include peer support networks, dementia advisers, or volunteer 'buddies'—there might even be a walking group Derek could join.

- Occupational therapists, who can advise on the use of assistive technology and minor adaptations to improve Derek's safety and independence, and help him to participate in exercise, leisure, and meaningful activity (College of Occupational Therapists 2011).

Rabinder's story

Rabinder is in his 60s and is living with chronic kidney disease. He failed to attend a recent hospital appointment for dialysis. When the administrator rang to speak to him, Rabinder answered the phone but then hung up. Claudia—a nurse on the dialysis care team—goes out to visit him to find out how he is.

When she gets to his house, Rabinder opens the door but refuses to let her in. He says he has decided that he wants to stop the dialysis and that he just wants to be left alone to die in peace. Claudia notices a strong smell of alcohol on his breath. She asks after his wife, Gurdeep, and Rabinder explains that she has had to go at short notice to Punjab for her mother's funeral. Rabinder looks very unkempt, and Claudia is concerned about his well-being. She asks if anyone else is looking after him, and he explains that he just wants to be on his own and shuts the door.

Claudia goes back to the office and is keen to get her manager's views on what should happen next.

What is our 'duty of care' here?

Rabinder has the right to refuse treatment if:

- He is 'competent';
- He has enough information to make the decision;
- He is making it voluntarily.

So, Claudia and her manager need to be absolutely confident that his competence has been assessed and that Rabinder has received and understood information about the implications of his choices.

Is Rabinder 'competent' to make this decision?

Just because Rabinder is refusing treatment which he needs to stay alive, it does not follow that he is 'incompetent'; this is the equivalent of making an 'unwise decision' under the MCA. However, the fact that he seems to be drinking heavily and may also be depressed does cast some doubt over Rabinder's competence. When Gurdeep returns, she will want to know what steps the team took to persuade her husband to continue with his treatment. Although this doesn't change Rabinder's right to refuse the treatment, it certainly increases the pressure on Claudia and her manager not to simply accept his refusal at face value.

What might the cultural and gender issues be here?

Recent evidence suggests that depression and alcohol use can be high within Sikh communities and that, for men in particular, there can be significant stigma attached to depression and other mental health issues (British Sikh Report 2018). It may be that Rabinder would prefer to speak to someone who shared his cultural background, or it may be that this would only intensify any feelings of shame; but either way, it will be important to be sensitive to his cultural and religious context.

Who else should be involved?

This is not a responsibility which Claudia, even with her manager's support, should take single-handedly: Rabinder's GP, his consultant, and a social worker attached to the team should meet to agree the best way forwards here. They might decide to make a referral to the alcohol and/or mental health team to get a specialist assessment of Rabinder's state of mind, if he can be persuaded to engage.

What is Claudia's emotional response to this?

All of this is likely to have an emotional impact on Claudia—this is perfectly natural and should not be suppressed: the law and good practice guidelines can take us only so far, and our emotional response can sometimes be a useful source of 'evidence' regarding how we might proceed. However, it is really important that we acknowledge the emotions we are feeling and seek to understand how they might shape our decision-making in relation to risk.

Guthrie (2018) has described this as the need to develop our 'Inner Supervisor', and become aware of the different thoughts and feelings we have about risks and rights, based on our professional self, our personal self, and the organisational culture in which we work. In this case, for example, Claudia's inner supervisor might reflect on the following different emotional responses she may be having:

Professional self: Claudia knows that Rabinder is putting his life at serious risk by refusing his dialysis treatment; even delaying it—should he later change his mind—may create further damage to the kidneys. The treatment has been working well so far, which increases her sense of frustration and disbelief.

Personal self: Claudia may have a number of personal emotional responses, based on her beliefs, and her own life experiences. She may, for example, hold strong views about suicide and assisted dying based on her religious beliefs; she may have had experiences of heavy drinking, depression, suicide, or people receiving successful treatment for similar conditions in her own life or amongst her family and friends.

Organisational culture: Claudia may be feeling anxious about the fact that Gurdeep will launch a complaint on her return, if Claudia fails to persuade Rabinder to resume his dialysis. Outcomes of past cases, or even investigations, her status in the organisation as relatively new in post, may all create anxiety for her.

If Claudia is able to reflect upon her different responses to Rabinder's situation, she may recognise that she feels pulled in different directions. Noticing this tension, and perhaps talking about it with a trusted colleague, manager or mentor might help her to identify the most important priorities and decide how to act.

Nursing people whose behaviour creates risk of harm

Balancing risks and rights, especially in communal settings, such as wards and care homes, is a day-to-day challenge for those nursing older people. As such settings include an increasing proportion of people with cognitive impairments, staff may find they are regularly responding to risks to self and others arising from behaviours such as aggression, 'wandering', agitation, sexual disinhibition, and persistent calling out.

Backhouse et al. (2017) spent many hours observing practice in four care (including two with nursing) homes. Although she did not witness any safeguarding issues, she nevertheless found that methods such as surveillance, positioning (and re-positioning), segregation, restrictions (such as locked doors and simple restraint), and forced care were in frequent use to manage risks. Often these were quite justifiable in the moment: usually they were used either where distraction and encouragement had failed and/or when risks were felt to be high and immediate. Nevertheless, she observed how 'non-standard actions', first used in response to crisis situations or one person's specific needs, can easily become 'established and routine practice, embedded in the setting as unquestioned usual practice' (p. 3). Although patient and staff safety was the primary driver, she found a grey area between this and the needs of 'organisational efficiency'—which is an increasing pressure as budgets tighten and staffing levels reduce.

She argues:

> Staff are being left with society's unresolved moral dilemma. The balance of individual freedom with personal risk taking and negative consequences of behaviour on other people is likely to have been present when the person was living in the community, and 'resolved' for the community by the person moving out of the community and into a residential setting. The dilemma still remains however behind closed doors; it is infrequently spoken about and is found in the internal experiences of both the staff and the residents.
>
> (p. 17)

There are no easy answers to these dilemmas; however, they should be reduced if we can better understand and seek to prevent high risk behaviours through more psychologically informed approaches.

If you are working in a care home or hospital where you think a person is being deprived of their liberty and this seems unavoidable, you should make an application for a Deprivation of Liberty Safeguards (DoLS) authorisation (SCIE 2017). However, first you should see if care could be provided in a less restrictive way: we spend the rest of the chapter discussing how you might go about this.

All behaviour—even where people are experiencing psychosis or serious cognitive impairment—has a function. A key message of Graham Stokes' (Stokes 2008) excellent and very readable book, "And still the music plays: stories of people with dementia", is that the behaviours of people with advanced dementia which we experience as challenging, puzzling, and irrational can be understood and managed effectively from a place of empathy.

For this to happen, we need to try and find out more about the person, their history, their personality prior to diagnosis, and their likes and dislikes. If we want to break the cycle of 'quick fixes', like doubling up staff, restraining or segregating someone (which may temporarily contain and manage the behaviour, but often intensify it and have a negative impact on everyone's well-being), we need to behave like a detective.

Stokes tells the story of Mr G, who has been placed on a specialist dementia unit. The manager of the unit asked Stokes for advice on how to manage Mr G's 'unpredictably violent' behaviour. He set up a log for staff to record incidents of violence, and, after just 9 days, 47 incidents had been recorded. However, the log revealed a clear pattern—the incidents were not as 'unpredictable' as previously thought: almost all were in response to Mr G receiving intimate care from staff. Typically, he would wet or soil himself, then become aggressive with staff who found and tried to change him.

Stokes spoke to Mrs G to build a picture of her husband. He had never had any issues using the toilet at home, before moving into the unit the month before. He had always been a proud and insular man, never really a 'people person', but a dedicated school teacher who loved to impart learning, and an avid gardener, who would spend hours alone in the garden.

Stokes felt that the layout of the unit, in which it was impossible to see or recognise the toilets from the communal lounge where Mr G often sat, was not helping matters. He figured that Mr G was too proud to ask where the toilets were, yet when asked if he needed the toilet (or discovered to have wet or soiled himself), he felt this was an affront to his dignity and he responded aggressively.

A care plan was designed, drawing on what had been learned about what makes Mr G tick:

- Every two hours, Mr G was to be approached, but with no initial mention of the word 'toilet'; staff were to ask his advice about the sensory garden: did the shrubs need pruning or the lawn mowing (thereby blending both his status as teacher and his love of gardening)?
- They would take him out to the gardens, passing the toilets on the way and saying casually, "I'm nipping into the toilets as we might be in the garden for a while, do you want to go too?"
- After going to the toilet, they would then take Mr G to the garden, saying how grateful they were for his help. When he got into the garden, he came 'alive', and a gentler, more peaceful air surrounded him' (Stokes 2018, p. 215).

The care plan was successful for the next 19 months, until Mr G became too frail to walk, but at this point he accepted the care he needed and did not resist. Despite his very short memory, this may well have been due to the manner of staff and the way they approached him: where previously they had been (understandably) afraid of him, 'he had gained the respect of staff who had seen another side of him, a side that warranted respect' (Stokes 2018, p. 216) (Box 4.1).

Box 4.1 Key principles and tips for working with people whose behaviour creates risk of harm

- Record and analyse the behaviour, looking for any patterns:
    - Are there particular times of day when the behaviour occurs, or certain triggers for it—like receiving personal care?
    - Does the person respond differently to men, women, people in uniforms, or different types of settings (in another of Stoke's stories, the colour in which a room was painted was bringing back painful memories for someone)?
    - What are the *possible* explanations for the behaviour?
- Find out as much as you can about the person from family, friends, or by asking them during calmer moments (if they are non-verbal, sometimes looking through a selection of photos or leafing through magazines might give some clues):
    - What did they used to do—for work, leisure, what roles did they play within this, what passions did they have?
    - How would others describe their personality?
    - Any known (or suspected) losses, traumas, and experiences of abuse: reliving these experiences as though they happened yesterday may explain violent reactions to personal care, constantly unsettled and distressed behaviour, etc.
- Put this information together to come up with a consistent care plan to pilot.
    - If we have a sense of what might be making the person feel unsafe (and hence triggering behaviours), how can we draw on our knowledge of them in order to make them feel safe?
    - For example, rather than two people in uniform bathing someone who often resists, can we turn bath time into a relaxing time, using scents, sounds, and lights that the person finds calming, based on what we know about them?
    - In the true spirit of piloting something, we should record and analyse the implementation and impact of the care plan. We may not get it right first time but, like a detective giving up one line of enquiry to pursue another, we should learn from this and move on, rather than abandon all hope of finding an approach that works. If we are to manage risks effectively, we need to be allowed and allow ourselves to take some risks along the way.

Summary of key messages

There are a number of key messages running through this chapter:

- We need to look beyond the risk of physical harm when assessing risks; risks to social and emotional well-being, especially where autonomy is reduced, are often at least as important for older people.
- We need to collaborate with older people and their families if we are to effectively assess, weigh up, and manage risks.

- We can enable older people to 'take (back) control' by giving them information, confidence, and support to problem-solve. They will then work to balance the risks themselves, in order to do the things that matter to them.
- We need to take time to try and understand the purpose of behaviour which seems puzzling; if we can do this, we can prevent many 'high risk' behaviours.
- We have a key role to play in challenging assumptions that older people 'need to be protected', and risk management practices which have become the norm, often for the sake of organisational efficiency.
- We—and everyone else involved—will have an emotional response to dilemmas of risks and rights. We need to be aware of our own responses and how they might shape our judgement, and encourage others to express their hopes and fears too.

References

Alzheimer's Society (2018). Which sections of the Mental Health Act are relevant to dementia? Accessed 31/05/2018 from www.alzheimers.org.uk/get-support/legal-and-financial/which-sections-mental-health-act-are-relevant-dementia

Andrews, J. (2017). '"Wandering" and dementia.' *British Journal of Community Nursing* 22(7), 322–323.

Andrews, N., Gabbay, J., le May, A., et al. (2015). *Developing Evidence Enriched Practice in Health and Social Care with Older People.* York: Joseph Rowntree Foundation.

Backhouse, T., Penhale, B., Gray, R., et al. (2017). 'Questionable practices despite good intentions: coping with risk and impact from dementia-related behaviours in care homes.' *Ageing & Society* 1–26. doi: 10.1017/S0144686X17000368.

Blood, I., Copeman, I. & Pannell, J. (2016). *Hearing the Voices of Older People in Wales: What Helps and Hinders as We Age?* Cardiff: Social Services Improvement Agency.

Blood, I. & Guthrie, L. (2018). *Supporting Older People Using Attachment-Informed and Strengths-Based Approaches.* York: Jessica Kingsley Publishers.

Blood, I. & Litherland, R. (2015). *Care Home Whispers: Listening to the voices of Older People living in Gloucestershire Care Homes.* Gloucester: Age UK Gloucestershire. www.ageuk.org.uk/gloucestershire/information-advice/care-home-whispers/

British Sikh Report (2018). 6th Annual British Sikh Report. www.britishsikhreport.org/wp-content/uploads/2018/05/British-Sikh-Report-2018.pdf

Clarke, C.L., Wilkinson, H., Keady, J., et al. (2011). *Risk Assessment and Management for Living Well with Dementia.* London: Jessica Kingsley Publishers.

College of Occupational Therapists (2011). Occupational Therapists help those with dementia and their carers. Occupational Therapy Evidence: Factsheet.

Finlayson, S. (2015). *Stop Worrying About Risk.* Blog: The Centre for Welfare Reform. www.centreforwelfarereform.org/library/by-az/stop-worrying-about-risk.html

Gardiner, S., Glogowska, M., Stoddart, C., et al. (2017). 'Older people's experiences of falling and perceived risk of falls in the community: a narrative synthesis of qualitative research.' *International Journal of Older People Nursing* 2017, 12e12151. doi: 10.1111/opn.12151

Guthrie, L. (2018). *Risks, Rights, Values and Ethics: Frontline Briefing.* Dartington: Research in Practice for Adults.

Horton, K. (2007). 'Gender and the risk of falling: A sociological approach.' *Journal of Advanced Nursing* 57(1), 69–76.

McMillan, L., Booth, J., Currie, K., et al. (2014). '"Balancing risk" after fall-induced hip fracture: The older person's need for information.' *International Journal of Older People Nursing* 9, 249–257. doi: 10.1111/opn.12028

Morgan, S. & Andrews, N. (2016). 'Positive risk-taking: From rhetoric to reality.' *The Journal of Mental Health Training, Education and Practice* 11(2), 122–132.

Parliamentary and Health Service Ombudsman (2016). *A Report of Investigations into Unsafe Discharge from Hospital.* London: Parliamentary and Health Service Ombudsman.

Robinson, L., Hutchings, D., Corner, L., et al. (2007). 'Balancing rights and risks: Conflicting perspectives in the management of wandering in dementia.' *Health, Risk & Society* 9(4), 389–406.

SCIE (Social Care Institute for Excellence) (2017). Deprivation of Liberty Safeguards (DoLs) at a glance, At a Glance 43. Accessed 31/05/2018 from www.scie.org.uk/mca/dols/at-a-glance

Stokes, G. (2008). *And Still the Music Plays–Stories of people with dementia.* London: Hawker Publications Ltd.

Vallelly, S., Evans, S., Fear, T., et al. (2006) *Opening Doors to Independence–A Longitudinal Study Exploring the Contribution of Extra Care Housing to the Care and Support of Older People with Dementia.* Bristol: University of the West of England/ Housing Corporation/Housing 21.

5 Staying healthy in older age

Andrée le May and Heather Fillmore Elbourne

Introduction

Healthy ageing is largely about having a healthy lifestyle. Ageing brings with it the likelihood of organ and system deterioration with the related challenges of reduced functionality, frailty, multimorbidity, and polypharmacy. Reducing the impact of age-related decline is important, not only to individuals but also to society. The World Health Organization (WHO) (2015) defined healthy ageing as:

> The process of developing and maintaining the functional ability that enables well-being in older age.

This definition seems to emphasise the functional elements of ageing, but it is important to consider all factors—social, physical, and psychological that impact on successful ageing, so you may find it useful to keep Katz et al.'s (2011) model in mind (see Chapter 2) as you read on. This chapter suggests some ways of staying healthy in older age.

Older people have not always been the target for health promotion messages, in fact they have been a relatively neglected group until WHO in 2001 stressed the importance of a healthy lifestyle to people at *all* stages of life (Golinowska et al. 2016). Before then it was felt that older age would not be a time when changes to lifelong habits were likely to occur and prompting them might, undesirably, disturb an older person's sense of peace and well-being (Golinowska et al. 2016). Views and attitudes have altered considerably since then, with older people being increasingly encouraged to take responsibility for their health in the hope of making older age a more positive and healthier experience.

Maintaining health and preventing its deterioration is an essential part of high-quality nursing, and it is with this in mind that we focus here on what nurses can encourage older people to do to enable them to stay in the best possible, all-round health. Whilst choosing how to maintain physical, mental, and spiritual health is an individual decision—older people cannot be treated simply as a homogenous group (www.theguardian.com/society/2015/mar/31/sod-70-hate-being-elderly), there is now sufficient evidence to show which lifestyle choices impact positively on health and well-being at all stages of older age. Some of these activities are detailed here.

Health promotion strategies in older age have three key aims: maintaining and increasing functional capacity, maintaining or improving self-care, and stimulating social interactions (Golinowska et al. 2016). If we are to achieve these broad aims we need to target key areas susceptible to improvement such as immobility and falls, feelings of reduced independence or actual dependence, loneliness and depression, cognitive decline and memory loss, and insomnia (see also Chapters 6 and 7). Lessening the burden of any of these will positively influence health and well-being. We focus below on three evidence-based strategies—increasing exercise, maintaining mental agility, and continuing social interaction that have this potential, and how these strategies can be enabled by social prescribing, motivational interviewing, and the use of assistive technologies.

Increasing exercise

We have known for some time that exercise, sometimes much less than we expect (Warburton and Bredin 2016), is beneficial to health. Warburton et al.'s (2006) narrative review confirmed several health benefits of exercise in older age including reductions in falls and muscle wasting, improved cardiovascular health, reduced risk of certain long-term conditions e.g. type-2 diabetes and some cancers, and improvements in some bone and joint conditions such as osteoporosis and osteoarthritis. Improvements in mental health have also been reported but seem to be more nuanced with inconsistent findings about the effectiveness of exercise in reducing feelings of depression (e.g. Bridle et al. 2012, Mura and Carta 2013; Underwood et al. 2013). However, there appears more consistency when we focus on cognitive decline. Northey et al.'s recent review (2017) concludes that physical exercise improves cognitive function in people aged 50+ regardless of their cognitive status, and Panza et al.'s (2018) review shows that exercise can delay decline in cognitive function for people with Alzheimer's disease. Recently, in a systematic review and meta-analysis Gheysen et al. (2018) reported positive effects on cognitive function when physical exercises were combined with cognitive exercises.

Exercises undertaken in groups may decrease social isolation and increase feelings of well-being (Hwang et al. 2016) and as you can see from Audrey's story in Appendix 1 also have a positive impact on insomnia. But despite numerous public health campaigns (e.g. Age UK's Fit as a Fiddle campaign between 2007 and 2012; Active Ageing Canada www.activeagingcanada.ca/) and readily available exercise guidelines/factsheets/films for older people advocating the advantages of exercising (e.g. www.nhs.uk/live-well/exercise/physical-activity-guidelines-older-adults/ and www.nhs.uk/Livewell/fitness/Documents/older-adults-65-years.pdf and www.csp.org.uk/public-patient/keeping-active-and-healthy/staying-healthy-you-age/staying-strong-you-age/strength), inactivity remains common.

What stops and helps older people to exercise?

Whilst there are many reasons why people don't exercise (we all have them!) the literature suggests that there are some that are specific to older people. Bethancourt et al. (2014) asked 52 Americans aged between 66 and 78, in 4 focus groups, about barriers to and facilitators of undertaking exercise. They categorised the findings into four groups—intrapersonal factors (linked to physical and mental health and individual preferences), interpersonal factors, physical environment factors, and structural and organisational factors. The findings show the range of issues that impact on the acceptability of exercise and are useful for anyone planning to develop exercise activities for older people. For instance, physical health barriers included pain, risk of injury, and fear of falling; individual preferences highlighted boredom, dislike of gyms, fear of intimidation or embarrassment as barriers and being pushed too hard or not enough were given as interpersonal factors that were off-putting. As one might expect environment barriers included the terrain (hills and stairs, uneven pavements), weather, and parking. Structural and organisational barriers encompassed expense and programmes not being at the right level—either too challenging or not being challenging enough. Facilitators clustered around the recognition of health gains (including prevention and maintenance of long-term conditions, weight loss, and mood enhancement) as well as enjoyment, camaraderie, and social contact. In addition, low-cost, high-quality instructors providing engaging and flexible programmes also facilitated attendance.

> **Think about this ...**
>
> Ask three older people what they do to exercise, what they enjoy or dislike about what they do, and if they'd change their level of exercise and why they would change it or wouldn't? (See Box 5.1.). Ask them how the exercise pattern has changed over their lifetime?

How can older people be encouraged to exercise?

Nurses, especially those working in primary/community care settings, have an important role in identifying older people who are inactive and advising them about the benefits of exercise as well as appropriate levels of exercise (see the latest guidance from your country's Department of Health and Social Care, or equivalent). This advice should focus on them as individuals and how they might achieve their goals. NICE (2013 reviewed 2016) recommends that nurses give 'brief advice'[1] focused on the latest government guidelines, the individual's health status, current level of activity, and his/her preferences, goals, and motivations for exercise. Having made an initial assessment, the nurse could use motivational interviewing (see Chapter 4 and the RCN Supporting Behaviour Change programme (www.rcn.org.uk/clinical-topics/supporting-behaviour-change) as a technique to help in the planning of an exercise programme (and its evaluation) with the person and their partner or family if appropriate. Nurses should also supplement their advice with written leaflets or give useful, up-to-date weblinks.

It is still unusual for nurses to run, or be involved in, exercise programmes for older people but there are examples of such schemes e.g. Inokuchi et al.'s 2007 successful community-based scheme in Japan and London's King's College Hospital NHS Trust's 'ward work-out scheme' on its rehabilitation wards. You can read about the King's College Hospital programme, how they implemented it and their success, in their project report. (www.fons.org/Resources/Documents/Project%20Reports/41-ExerciseFinalNov2005.pdf).

> **Think about this ...**
>
> Collect some information about where you work.
>
>   Are there any exercise programmes for older people in your work-place or associated services? If so find out how older people get referred to them – or find out about

them? Ask around and see if nurses are involved in these sorts of programmes and see if you could attend a class or two? Ask if nurses are involved in writing NHS Exercise on Prescription for these classes.

(see Box 5.1)

Maintaining mental agility

Maintaining cognitive function and mental agility (cognitive health) is a very important aspect of healthy aging, and many 'tips' on how to do this are written in the popular literature and professional journals. For instance, not long ago Psychology Today (2014) published Eight Habits that Improve Cognitive Function: these were taking exercise, being open to new experiences, being curious and creative, making social connections, using mindfulness techniques, doing brain-training exercises, getting sufficient sleep, and reducing long-term stress (www.psychologytoday.com/intl/blog/the-athletes-way/201403/eight-habits-improve-cognitive-function). Other similar lists can be found by searching the internet e.g. the Canadian website Memory Fitness® (www.memoryfitness.ca/) advocates physical activity, cognitive exercises, and social interaction; NICE's (2016) guidance on 'Older people: independence and mental wellbeing' recommends many group and individual pursuits ranging from singing to reading with children in schools—these all enhance social interactions as well as promoting new experiences (www.nice.org.uk/guidance/ng32/chapter/Recommendations#onetoone-activities).

More specifically Kelly et al.'s (2014) systematic review and meta-analysis showed that cognitive training improved older people's ability to undertake cognitive tasks and some aspects of memory (e.g. face-name recall, immediate recall) but that more work was required to determine if general mental stimulation positively impacts on cognitive and everyday functioning. More recently Belleville et al. (2018) showed that memory training can improve memory in older people with amnesic mild cognitive impairment (aMCI). Savulich et al. (2017) have developed a new memory training app 'Game Show' which has shown positive results when used by people with aMCI. Other similarly innovative technological developments are being evaluated or used to increase our knowledge about how older people's brains function (e.g. the Brain-Changer project www.bdi.ox.ac.uk/news/new-app-to-improve-dementia-diagnosis-launched which is collecting information about cognitive function while people without dementia play certain games on their phones—any person over 18 can join so why not have a look).

Nurses come into contact with older people in almost every aspect of their work and so are in a good position to advice older people and/or their families and carers about ways to keep cognitively healthy. As you can see from the eight tips above there are a variety of very simple things that older people can be encouraged to do to improve their cognitive abilities, ranging from making sure they get enough sleep and physical exercise and eat well to trying daily brain-training exercises or other intellectually stimulating activities. As with encouraging someone to exercise physically encouraging cognitive exercise will necessitate individual discussions and goal setting. Motivational interviewing might be an important strategy to use in conjunction with written/electronic information and advice. One useful internet site for people with mild to moderate cognitive impairment is the Age UK's Maintenance Cognitive Stimulation Therapy (MCST) website www.ageuk.org.uk/our-impact/programmes/maintenance-cognitive-stimulation-therapy-mcst/.

Think about this ...

Collect some information about your local facilities.

Find out about clubs and classes that older people might attend in your geographical area. See if your local GP/family doctor surgery has a list of nearby ones? Find out also if there are third sector/charitable organisations who provide places for people to meet and chat or learn new activities and skills. See if you can visit one and see what goes on.

Continuing social interaction

Continuing to have social interactions in older age is an important factor in reducing social isolation and loneliness as well as maintaining mental well-being and independence (NICE 2016). Loneliness and social isolation are related but not the same (Age UK 2015), and a person can feel lonely without being socially isolated and vice versa. In their evidence review on loneliness Age UK (2015) defines loneliness and social isolation as follows:

> Loneliness can be understood as an individual's personal, subjective sense of lacking desired affection, closeness, and social interaction with others. Although loneliness has a social aspect, it is also defined by an individual's subjective emotional state. Loneliness is more dependent on the quality than the number of relationships.
> Social isolation refers to a lack of contact with family or friends, community involvement, or access to services.
>
> (p. 3)

Age UK (2015) present some stark facts about older people's lives and the impact of loneliness on their health and well-being. For instance, 49% of people aged over 65 in the United Kingdom say that television or pets are their main form of company, 41% of people aged 65+ in the United Kingdom feel out of touch with the pace of modern life, and 12% say they feel cut off from society (TNS Loneliness Survey for Age UK, April 2014). The impact of loneliness may be as harmful to health as smoking 15 cigarettes a day (Holt-Lunstad et al. 2010). Age UK also collated evidence of factors that impact on loneliness suggesting that some people from certain groups seem to be more at risk of being isolated and lonely as they get older than others e.g. older women, informal carers, people living on low incomes, people from ethnic minority groups, and gay men and lesbians.

What can be done to diminish feelings of loneliness?

The literature suggests that things can be done to lessen loneliness at an individual or group level. At an individual level these may include using a befriending service where a volunteer visits regularly e.g. through the Royal Voluntary Service (www.royalvoluntaryservice. org.uk), or developing telephone/letter friends who call/write regularly e.g. Silver Line offers a Silver Line Friend for regular weekly telephone calls and Silver Letters (www.thesilverline. org.uk). Under the former UK Prime Minister's new Loneliness Strategy announced in October 2018 postal workers are going to be able to call on lonely people to check how they are and to try to link them with support networks (www.gov.uk/government/news/pm-launches-governments-first-loneliness-strategy)–a similar scheme is in operation in France (www.theguardian.com/world/2018/nov/23/care-package-french-postal-workers-helping-lonely-older-people). Older people are increasingly competent and comfortable using the internet and mobile phone technology as a medium for communication enabling contact to be easily made with faraway family and friends; new friends can also be made through chat rooms for those unable to leave their homes. Silversurfers, a long-standing website for older people, offers advice on how to find the best chat room (www.silversurfers.com/best-of-the-web/technology-best-of-the-web/best-senior-chat-rooms-sites-for-over-50s-60s/).

At a group level there are many activities that older people can undertake ranging from volunteering, to taking classes for learning new skills and knowledge, to trips to see new places. For those who are perhaps less active and require more care there are day centres and lunch clubs run by health- and social-care services as well as many charitable organisations. There are also activities emerging for specific groups of people who are often socially isolated. Probably the best known one of these is 'Men in Sheds' (https://menssheds.org.uk/) which was designed to provide community spaces where men 'connect, converse, and create' together rather than individually in their sheds. Age UK (www.ageuk.org.uk), the United Kingdom's largest charity for older people, has local offices across the United Kingdom and is a good source of information that nurses can use to refer their patients to. Similar sorts of charitable organisations can be found across the world e.g. HelpAge Canada (https://helpagecanada.ca). The UK Campaign to End Loneliness website has a series of case studies describing ways through which loneliness can be alleviated (https://campaign-toendloneliness.org/guidance/theoretical-framework).

Again, nurses play an important part in pointing older people towards facilities for promoting social interaction. Find out what's going on near where you work or live so you have the information to hand. Motivational interviewing (see above and Chapter 4) and social prescribing might be two useful strategies to use if you are advising an older person or their family about increasing social interactions and decreasing loneliness (see also Chapter 6).

Think about this ...

Nurses also need to be aware of some of the many ways that loneliness can manifest, for instance a colleague of mine (AlM) told me a story about a primary care/practice nurse who noticed her patients with leg dressings kept coming back to her when they could manage their dressings themselves. She realised that they kept coming back because they were lonely and valued the interaction that having a dressing entailed so she decided to start a Leg Club where they could meet each other independently of having their dressing changed. Their overall wellbeing improved!

See here for more information about Leg Clubs www.legclub.org/

Can you think of similar circumstances? Ask your colleagues and mentors if they have any similar experiences.

Social prescribing

Social prescribing is a new trendsetter steeped in optimism in that it is thought to have the potential to improve people's health and well-being and cut health- and social-care costs (Kenkre and Howarth 2018). Social prescribing is defined as:

> A means of enabling GPs, nurses and other primary care professionals to refer people to a range of local, non-clinical services. Recognising that people's health is determined primarily by a range of social, economic and environmental factors, social prescribing seeks to address people's needs in a holistic way. It also aims to support individuals to take greater control of their own health. Social prescribing schemes can involve a variety of activities which are typically provided by voluntary and community sector organisations. Examples include volunteering, arts activities, group learning, gardening, befriending, cookery, healthy eating advice and a range of sports.
>
> (King's Fund 2017: www.kingsfund.org.uk/publications/
> social-prescribing?gclid=EAIaIQobChMIpOOC6-uQ3wIV6Z3tCh2h-
> wozEAAYASAAEgLqvPD_BwE#what-is-it)

Although there is little evidence that social prescribing is effective yet (Bickerdike et al. 2017) it is being promoted by UK government policy (e.g. Loneliness Strategy 2018, www.gov.uk/government/news/pm-launches-governments-first-loneliness-strategy), with Canada following suit (www.cbc.ca/news/canada/ottawa/social-prescribing-loneliness-health-problems-1.4833088), and is positively changing people's lives.

Think about this ...

Visit your local GP's/ family doctor's surgery and ask if they use social prescribing and if so who can "write" the prescriptions and what sort of activities are prescribed. If practice nurses are involved, try to talk to one of them about their experiences.

Boxes 5.1 and 5.2 show examples of nurses' involvement in social prescribing. In the first example Natasha Duke describes how she prescribed exercise for one of her patients whilst working as an advanced nurse practitioner in primary care, and in the second example Michelle Howarth, who leads the Nursing Social Prescribing Special Interest group (www.social prescribingnetwork.com/special-interest-groups), describes the impact of nature on a group of older people.

Box 5.1 Social prescribing in practice: encouraging exercise

Molly is a 62-year-old lady and attended her diabetes review with me. While doing all the routine tests for diabetes, I asked Molly 'Managing diabetes can be tough...is there anything you find particularly difficult?' These kinds of open questions can help diabetic patients talk about the challenges of eating a healthy diet and doing exercise.

I asked Molly to reflect on a typical day and was particularly listening to her attitude to exercise. Molly did not mention exercise in her day's routine at all.

I then asked Molly, 'It's really important to try to exercise for everyone, but especially if you have diabetes. Is this something you would like some help with?' Molly looked doubtful. 'I'm not very good at exercise, I just find it boring. I don't like going for walks and I hate swimming'. I asked her, 'Is there any kind of exercise you might like, anything at all?' Molly thought for a while and replied, 'I did like dancing when I was younger!' By listening to what appealed to Molly, I was able to inform her about a dance class at a local gym that she would be able to access at low cost, via the NHS 'Exercise on Prescription'. I informed her about the class, and then discussed any concerns that she might have about trying this. This component of the conversation is vital. The practitioner must explore barriers that could prevent the new idea from blossoming. Molly said she was worried about going alone, and she 'might feel silly being so old and going to a dance class'. These were real challenges for her considering the class. I replied, 'There's no pressure to decide today Molly, have a think about if this is something you'd be interested in. You could chat with a friend and see if they might like to go with you?'

The next consultation with Molly was three months later, where I raised the topic of the dance class again. She responded that she had talked with a friend and was open to the idea of the gym. I completed the relevant paperwork for Molly to take, and she rang her gym to organise her induction. Six months later, Molly had not only attended dance classes but also tried a few other classes due to the encouragement of her friend.

Box 5.2 Social prescription: the impact of nature on older people

We know that, globally, the population is getting older; the estimated growth has been described as 'unprecedented' (United Nations 2002). At a pathophysiological level, the impact of ageing is inevitable, and many people now live with co-morbid, long-term conditions. So, what is the role of nursing in supporting older people to live well and stay well? Ostensibly, nurses may have been subverted by a pathogenic approach to care through placing a precedence on the assessment of an older person's 'needs' rather than their 'assets'. In doing so, are we guilty of singling out the disease as champion and limiting the person as a patient? Enabling an older person's independence is a gift, but how we do this has often relied on a pathogenic approach, rather than one which looks to non-medical 'salutogenic' methods. In focusing on the individual's 'strengths' rather than 'needs' it is thought that older people will be more empowered to make lifestyle choices that are predicated on their passions rather than their ailments.

So, how can nurses use an asset-based, person-centred approach to empower older people? One solution could be the advent of 'social prescribing' which uses non-medical approaches to support people and communities to become resilient. As a process, social prescribing has received increasing recognition within the United Kingdom as an empowering social movement that can help connect people with alternative, non-medical approaches such as the arts, yoga, and nature. The latter, 'nature', presents a potent approach to enabling older people to live well and stay well through activities such as gardening, community allotments, or simply getting out and being in nature. In a recent study I was involved in (Howarth et al. 2018) older people were interviewed about their experiences of taking part in a gardening programme. A total of 30 older people between the ages of 65 and 90 took part in the gardening and reported benefits such as improved confidence, greater awareness of healthy food, improved social connection, and a renewed sense of meaning and purpose. Of particular note here, is the way in which nature-based activity such as gardening helped older people to reconnect and create relationships that extended beyond the gardening group.

The impact of social isolation is thought to be equivalent to smoking 15 cigarettes a day, yet, ironically, being outdoors in the fresh air can help improve physical activity such as heart rate and stress reduction, and, significantly for older people, can help people to reconnect. Could nurses use nature as a prescription? Arguably, we are not unaccustomed to this practice, in 1860, Florence Nightingale once wrote "I shall never forget the rapture of fever patients over a bunch of bright-coloured flowers... people say the effect is only on the mind. It is no such thing. The effect is on the body too". Contact with nature can help people re-establish well-being and can enhance a sense of belonging. So, isn't it time to revisit our prescription of 'nature', solicit it as a weapon against social isolation, and see the person rather than the patient.

Howarth M, Rogers M, Withnell N, and McQuarrie, C. 2018. Growing spaces: an evaluation of the mental health recovery programme using mixed methods. *Journal of Research in Nursing* 1-14.

United Nations. 2002. World population ageing: 1950-2050. Available from: www.un.org/esa/population/publications/worldageing19502050/ (accessed 21 May 2018)

Assistive technologies

The NIHR Dissemination Centre (2018) recently published a themed review on the use of assistive technologies for older people. In it (p. 5) they define assistive technology as:

> ... anything which helps people stay independent, manage their health or compensate for a disability. This includes everyday aids like walking frames or wheelchairs to more advanced digital technology like robots and the internet of things (where everyday household appliances and devices 'talk to' each other).
>
> (www.dc.nihr.ac.uk/themed-reviews/Help-at-home-WEB.pdf)

As the definition suggests the range of assistive technologies is diverse and includes some things that all nurses are familiar with such as monitoring, tracking or call devices (wearable alarm pendants or bracelets, movement sensors on chairs and beds, or home-installed sensors) linked to health/social-care professionals and carers, and remote monitoring of e.g. heart rate, blood pressure, and respiratory function which act as early warning systems of deteriorating health. Some people use household technologies such as specialist kitchen or bathroom devices to help them, and these too are classified as assistive technologies. Other more unusual technologies include using robots for lifting, delivering food, and taking vital signs—often as an adjunct to other carers (http://theconversation.com/nurses-of-the-future-must-embracehigh-tech-86042 and https://nurse.org/articles/nurse-robots-friend-or-foe/).

Think about this …

Anyone interested in thinking more about the impact – positive and negative, on older people of robots should read Laitinen et al's (2016) chapter on social robotics. http://roseproject.aalto.fi/images/publications/seibt225_Laitinen.pdf

Or for fun watch the film 'Robot & Frank' (2012).

How could robots influence an older person's wellbeing – either in a hospital or home setting?

Not all technology that is set up or purchased for older people is used or used properly. In Box 5.3 you can read an extract by Jenni Lynch from her PhD thesis showing how older people misuse or adapt their technologies. This sort of 'adaptation' means that not only is that person not receiving the best service and associated benefits, and so may be at risk, but also that any monitoring organisation/professional is receiving incorrect information and is unable to make accurate assessments of, or provide the right care to, the person with the technology. Sometimes this means that the professional carer thinks that a person is better or safer than they are. Nurses visiting or calling older people are in a good position to enquire about any assistive technologies being used and remind older people about the benefits of use whilst always checking if there are any problems or 'adaptations'. Encouraging older people to use their assistive technologies in the right way is a key part of a nurse's role, and motivational interviewing might be a useful persuasive technique to use (see Chapter 4 and the RCN Supporting Behaviour Change programme (www.rcn.org.uk/clinical-topics/supporting-behaviour-change) to ensure compliance.

Box 5.3 Experiences of using assistive technology: Jenni Lynch's research

Adapted from: Lynch, JK. Policy aspirations and practice in English telecare: a case study of story-lines and invisible work. University of Birmingham; 2015. http://ethos.bl.uk/OrderDetails.do?uin=uk.bl.ethos.675772

Examples of adaptation or misuse of the telecare equipment were frequently observed in this study and reported by participants. Mr and Mrs F were a couple in their 80s living in sheltered accommodation. Mr F was managing the majority of the care required by his wife who was living with dementia. The couple was supported by a community alarm system that connected a number of different sensors around their home. During a 12-month review visit by a telecare technician to check that the system was working correctly it became apparent that Mr F was switching off all electrical sockets every night rendering the sensors useless.

During an interview with Zainub, another service user over 80 years old who was living alone, she demonstrated how she had used a cushion to cover up the sensor that controlled her bedside lamp, as she was exasperated by the light being triggered every time she walked past it. Zainub's bed had been moved into the living room as she now struggled with the stairs and she explained that while the automatic light was appreciated at night, during the day this space was a hub of activity for her large family who frequently visited and often inadvertently activated the lamp. Thus, Zainub had to adapt the equipment to integrate it with the different aspects of her life—one of which led her to be grateful for the technology, another to be frustrated by it.

There were further similar examples of what might be described as involuntary non-use (Wyatt et al. 2002) of the assistive technology due to its poor integration with individual circumstances and lack of imparted knowledge about how equipment might be adjusted to work more effectively for service users. For example, Mrs C (90 years old and living alone) had a community alarm system and sensor-controlled lighting upstairs that would switch on lights when she got up in the night to go to the toilet. The telecare technician had been called to remove the sensors as Mrs C, who was dealing with deteriorating cognitive function, was increasingly distressed by the lights coming on as she couldn't remember why they were there and had begun to damage the sockets in efforts to turn them off. In a separate visit, Mrs W was also using the sensor-controlled lights and had tampered with the mechanism in an attempt to adjust the timer, but this caused it to stop working. As she hadn't reported the fault she had been managing without the lights for some time. In both these cases a lack of understanding of the workings of the devices led to their not being used—in the case of Mrs W this led to her realisation that she could cope without the equipment with few ill effects.

Wyatt S, Thomas G, and Terranova T. 2002. They came, they surfed, they went back to the beach, conceptualising use and non-use of the internet. In: Woolgar S (Ed.). *Virtual Society? Technology, Cyberbole, Reality*. Oxford University Press, Oxford, 23–40.

Summary of key messages

- Increasing exercise, maintaining mental agility, and continuing social interaction all have the potential to improve older people's health and well-being.
- Each of these activities can be undertaken individually or collectively.

- There are many influences on undertaking activities in older age, and nurses can play an important part in recognising these and helping, in conjunction with other members of the multidisciplinary team, to reduce barriers.
- Nurses, in all settings and roles, can advise older people and their families about ways to improve their health and well-being. To do this, nurses may use motivational interviewing or social prescribing.
- Many older people use assistive technologies to help them live more independently and to monitor their health more effectively, thus helping them to stay healthier. Nurses need to encourage the proper use of these technologies and be able to guide older people in their use or to experts who can help them.

Note

1 'verbal advice, discussion, negotiation or encouragement, with or without written or other support or follow-up; it can vary from basic advice to a more extended, individually focused discussion' NICE (2013).

References

Age UK. 2015. Evidence review: loneliness in later life. www.ageuk.org.uk/globalassets/age-uk/documents/reports-and-publications/reports-and-briefings/health--wellbeing/rb_june15_lonelines_in_later_life_evidence_review.pdf

Belleville S, Hudon C, Bier N, et al. 2018. MEMO+: efficacy, durability and effect of cognitive training and psychosocial intervention in individuals with mild cognitive impairment. *Journal of the American Geriatrics Society* 66(4):655–663.

Bethancourt H, Rosenberg D, Beatty T, et al. 2014. Barriers to and facilitators of physical activity program use among older adults. *Clinical Medicine and Research* 12(1–2):10–20.

Bickerdike L, Booth A, Wilson P, et al. 2017. Social prescribing: less rhetoric and more reality. A systematic review of the evidence. *BMJ Open* 7:e013384.

Bridle C, Spanjers K, Patel S, et al. 2012. Effect of exercise on depression severity in older people: systematic review and meta-analysis of randomised controlled trials. *British Journal of Psychiatry* 201:180–185.

Gheysen F, Poppe L, DeSmet A, et al. 2018. Physical activity to improve cognition in older adults: can physical activity programs enriched with cognitive challenges enhance the effects? A systematic review and meta-analysis. *International Journal of Behavioral Nutrition and Physical Activity* 15:63.

Golinowska S, Groot W, Baji P, and Pavlova M. 2016. Health promotion targeting older people. *BMC Health Services Research* 16(Suppl 5):345.

Holt-Lunstad J, Smith TB, and Layton JB. 2010. Social relationships and mortality risk: a meta-analytic review. *PLoS Medicine* 7:7.

Hwang J, Wang L, and Jones C. 2016. Tackling social isolation and loneliness through community exercise programs for seniors. *UBC Medical Journal* 8(1):38–39.

Inokuchi S, Matsusaka N, Hayashi T, et al. 2007. Feasibility and effectiveness of a nurse-led community exercise programme for prevention of falls among frail elderly people: a multi-centre controlled trial. *Journal of Rehabilitation Medicine* 39(16):479–485.

Katz J, Holland C, Peace S, et al. 2011. *A better life: what older people with high support needs value.* Joseph Rowntree Foundation, York.

Kelly M, Loughrey D, Lawlor B, et al. 2014. The impact of cognitive training and mental stimulation on cognitive and everyday functioning of healthy older adults: a systematic review and meta-analysis. *Ageing Research Reviews* 15:28–43.

Kenkre J, and Howarth M. 2018. Guest editorial: social prescribing. *Journal of Research in Nursing* 23(8):640–645.

Laitinen A, Niemelä M, and Pirhonen J. 2016. Social robotics, elderly care, and human dignity: a recognition-theoretical approach. In: Seibt J, Nørskov M, and Schack Andersen S (Eds.). *What social robots can and should do: proceedings of robophilosophy 2016.* http://roseproject.aalto.fi/images/publications/seibt225_Laitinen.pdf

Mura G, and Carta M. 2013. Physical activity in depressed elderly. A systematic review. *Clinical Practice and Epidemiology in Mental Health* 9:125–135.

NICE. 2013. Physical activity: brief advice for adults in primary care. Public health guideline [PH44] National Institute for Health and Care Excellence, London.

NICE. 2016. Mental wellbeing and independence for older people. Quality standard [QS137] National Institute for Health and Care Excellence, London.

Northey JM, Cherbuin N, Pumpa KL, et al. 2017. Exercise interventions for cognitive function in adults older than 50: a systematic review with meta-analysis. *British Journal of Sports Medicine* 52(3): 154–160.

Panza GA, Taylor BA, MacDonald HV, et al. 2018. Can exercise improve cognitive symptoms of Alzheimer's disease? A meta-analysis. *International Journal of the American Geriatrics Society* 66(3):487–495.

Savulich G, Piercy T, Fox C, et al. 2017. Cognitive training using a novel memory game on an iPad in Patients with Amnestic Mild Cognitive Impairment (aMCI). *International Journal of Neuropsychopharmacology* 20(8):624–633.

Underwood M, Lamb SE, Eldridge S, et al. 2013. Exercise for depression elderly residents of care homes: a cluster-randomised controlled trial. *The Lancet* 382 (9886):41–49.

Warburton D, Nicol C, and Bredin S. 2006. Health benefits of physical activity. *Canadian Medical Association Journal* 174(6):801–809.

Warburton D, and Bredin S. 2016. Reflections on physical activity and health: what should we recommend? *Canadian Journal of Cardiology* 32(4):495–504.

WHO. 2015. World report on ageing and health. Luxembourg.

6 Common difficulties experienced by older people

Khim Horton

Introduction

People aged 65 or more make up about 17% of the population in England, and this group is more likely to utilise more than one sixth of some health- and social-care resources (Health and Social Care Information Centre, HSCIC 2014). There are now 11.8 million people aged 65 or over in the United Kingdom, of these 1.6 million people are aged 85 or over (Age UK 2017). According to the Health Survey for England (2015) 21% of men and 30% of women aged 65 and over required help with at least one Activity of Daily Living and 22% and 33%, respectively, needed help with at least one Instrumental Activity of Daily Living (IADL). Furthermore, an estimated 4 million older people in the United Kingdom (36% of people aged 65-74 and 47% of those aged 75+) have a limiting long-standing illness (Age UK 2017). It is therefore vital that nurses and other health-care professionals are familiar with common difficulties experienced by older people. Although problems such as incontinence, loss of mobility, falls, delirium, cognitive decline, cognitive impairment, and pain, commonly known as the 'geriatric syndromes', do not affect every older person, it is important that nurses have some knowledge and understanding about common difficulties experienced by older people to provide competent and compassionate care. Some older people may experience one or more of these difficulties, and these may change over time. In this chapter, I have chosen to focus on some of these common dificulties, which are inter-related— falls, urinary incontinence (UI), pain, reduced mobility, and physical activity and loneliness. Recent sources of the best evidence to help inform the nursing care of older people have been included.

Falls

It is commonly known that people aged 65 or more have the highest risk of falling (Dollard et al. 2014; National Institute for Health and Care Excellence (NICE) 2015a). About 30% of this age group and living at home will experience at least one fall a year (NICE 2013a). In England alone, this approximates 2.5 million people (NICE 2015a). The risk of falling increases to 50% of those aged over 80 who are either at home or in residential care (NICE 2015b; Royal College of Physicians, RCP 2015). It is estimated that the cost of falls to the National Health Service (NHS) is more than £2 billion per year (Snooks et al. 2011); this can have detrimental impact on productivity costs such as carer time and absence (Tian et al. 2013).

Most falls do not result in serious injury, but annually approximately 5% of older people living in the community who fall experience a fracture or need hospitalisation (RCP 2015). Falls are the largest cause of emergency hospital admissions for older people, and significantly impact on long-term outcomes, e.g. being a major precipitant of people moving from their own home to long-term nursing or residential care (Department of Health, DH 2012). For people living in the community, falls represent over half of hospital admissions for accidental injury, particularly hip fracture. Half of those with hip fracture never regain their former level of function and one in five die within three months (RCP 2015). Older people with multiple acute and chronic health problems are the group most vulnerable to falling.

By contrast, care home residents are among those at highest risk of falling and of sustaining injury as a result of falling. It is estimated that just over half the population of care home residents will suffer at least one fall per year and about 20 percent of all hip fractures occur in this group, even though only 3% of older people in England reside in care homes (RCP 2012). Up to 40% of ambulance call-outs to homes for people aged 65 or more are related to falls (Snook et al. 2011).

In hospital settings, in-patient falls are the most commonly reported patient safety incident with about 240,000 in-patient falls reported from hospitals and mental health units in England and Wales annually (RCP 2015). Public Health England highlighted that around 255,000 falls-related emergency hospital admissions in England among patients aged 65 and over occur each year (Fenton 2017). The cost implications cannot be underestimated with fragility fractures costing the United Kingdom an estimated £4.4 billion, of which 25% is for social care (Fenton 2017). The actual costs are likely to be higher taking into account the cost of additional health, social, and residential care that is often needed following discharge from hospital (Tian et al. 2013).

Given that inpatient falls are the most commonly reported patient safety incident with more than 250,000 reported in hospital trusts in England every year (that is over 700 a day), inpatient falls pose a major concern for NHS care providers as a marker of care quality (RCP 2014a). Worryingly, evidence from the National Hip Fracture Database (RCP 2014b) indicated more than 2,500 inpatient hip fractures were recorded in the year 2012–13. Outcomes for patients are not encouraging; mortality within one month is approximately 10%, and only 10% of patients who fracture a hip in a hospital fall will regain their previous levels of mobility. As people aged over 65 account for more than half of inpatient bed days in the NHS (HSCIC 2014), and the likelihood of longer hospital stay (Poteliakhoff and Thompson 2011; Cornwell et al. 2012; Foundation Trust Network 2012; Imison et al. 2012; NHS Improvement 2017), there is an urgent need to minimise any harm arising from inpatient falls as well as minimising deficiencies in usual care.

A national audit commissioned by the Healthcare Quality Improvement Partnership and conducted by the RCP involved NHS Trusts in England and Wales during May 2015 provides a snapshot of the organisational and clinical perspectives (RCP 2015); it indicated that although nearly all NHS hospital trusts have fall prevention policies, there was no association between what the policies included and what actually happened when a patient was admitted to hospital. This raises the importance of ensuring that such policies are embedded into practice.

A follow-up audit in 2017 by the RCP also found that only 19% of patients had their lying and standing blood pressure (BP) recorded (RCP 2017). This is a key concern since some patients may suffer from postural hypotension which increases their risk of falling. More could be done by making sure that older people are adequately hydrated and have their medication reviewed and modified (RCP 2017). It was recommended that hospital trusts could use the RCP clinical practice tool on how to take lying and standing BP to standardise practice (RCP 2017).

The impact of falls on older people, their family, and health and social care needs to be recognised. Not only do falls affect the quality of life on the individual, but they can also impact on older people's independence and morbidity and even cause death (Scheffer et al. 2008; World Health Organization 2008). For an older person with dementia, the gradual loss of safe mobility and ability to perform self-care as well as the inability to perceive risk increases their risk of falling (Ramaswamy and Jones 2012). A multidisciplinary approach to manage this difficulty is necessary; this may include referrals to an occupational therapist or physiotherapist for advice about equipment and adaptations to aid mobility and home environmental modifications to make living conditions safer.

An older person should receive a multifactorial risk assessment if they report: (a) two or more falls in the past 12 months, (b) seeking medical attention with a fall, and (c) difficulty with walking or balance (British Geriatrics Society 2016a). Older people should be encouraged to report all falls to their general practitioner (GP), so that risk factors can be identified and addressed (NICE 2013b).

There are no single or easily defined interventions which are shown to reduce falls making it challenging to tackle falls as patients vary as much as care settings (RCP 2015, 2017). The multiple causes of falls in older people compound any approach by health- and social-care providers to reduce falls. Any effort to prevent falls during acute illness involves interventions to change intrinsic patient-level risk factors while adapting their daily care requirements to anticipate and ameliorate the consequences of these risks (RCP 2014a). However, research has shown that multiple interventions performed by the multidisciplinary team and tailored to the individual patient can reduce falls by 20%–30% (RCP 2014a).

From a nursing perspective, caring for older people experiencing difficulties in relation to falls and managing their care in accordance to workable policies can be challenging. Policies in fall prevention interventions may include ensuring that those aged 65 or more (and those over 50 at particular risk) have a lying and standing BP and actions taken if there is a significant drop in BP on standing, and have a medication review looking particularly for medications likely to increase risks of falling (RCP 2015). Inadequate physiological response to such postural changes can lead to an abnormally large drop in BP; this is especially common in older people (O'Riordan et al. 2017). The measurement of lying and standing BP usually takes only 5–10 minutes, but only 19% of patients had this recorded (RCP 2017). Some hospitals managed to record this in most appropriate patients, and this is a clear area where hospitals can improve. O'Riordan et al. (2017) and Windsor et al. (2016) provide further information on this measurement.

A more structured approach involves risk assessment. NICE states that every patient aged 65 or more in hospital should be deemed to be at risk regardless of whether they have had a fall or not and that using risk prediction tools should be discouraged as none of the published studies on risk prediction tools yield more than 70% sensitivity (RCP 2015).

Nurses need to recognise the important role families and carers have in supporting older people who experience a fall. Therefore, involving family members and carers in the decision-making process about prevention, treatment, and care is critical, especially for those with dementia or delirium who are at high risk of falls in hospitals (RCP 2015).

Key points on falls

- About 30% of people aged 65 or more and living at home will experience at least one fall a year.
- Every patient aged 65 or more in hospital should be deemed to be at risk regardless of whether they have had a fall or not.
- NICE (2013b) specifically recommended that Falls Risk Screening Tools are not used in hospital.
- A drop in BP on standing may increase a person's risk of falling. Therefore, anyone aged 65 or more should have their lying and standing BP assessed and monitored if necessary.
- Medication review is recommended, especially those that are likely to increase the risk of falling.
- People with incontinence should have a continence plan. Incontinence and falls may be linked.
- People aged 65 or more should have a visual impairment assessment.

Urinary incontinence

Although UI is not life threatening, its impact on individuals living with this difficulty and on the health service cannot be underestimated. Sadly, many people with bladder and bowel incontinence experience this problem in silence, and are too embarrassed to seek help (RCP 2011). According to Age UK (2017), there are around 3.2 million people over 65 living with UI in the United Kingdom; findings from epidemiological studies show that about a third of older women aged 65 or more experience incontinence compared to one in seven older men of the same age group (Martin et al. 2006), and the prevalence increases with age (NICE 2013c). The prevalence of UI among those aged 40 or more is about 34% in women and 14% in men (Martin et al. 2006). It is estimated that more than 50% of care home residents have UI (Saxer et al. 2008). Studies have shown that UI affects one third of women, with the prevalence increasing with age. The British Geriatrics Society (2016b) estimated that problems with bladder control are common with two in five women aged 60 or more. Data also revealed that slight to moderate incontinence is more common in younger women, with moderate and severe incontinence mostly affecting older women (RCP 2011).

Suffice it to say, if not identified, assessed, and treated, undiagnosed UI can be costly to the NHS (Williams et al. 2005; Wagg et al. 2007; Thirugnanasothy 2010) and also to the person with incontinence if they are self-funding continence products. This problem also has a considerable personal cost to the individual and their family in terms of their quality of life.

Normal ageing processes that impact upon continence in older people include reduced sensitivity in neurological pathways between the bladder and the brain resulting in older people being unaware of the need to void their bladder until their bladder is 90% full, compared to younger adults, whose bladders register the need to go when they are 50% full (Nazarko 2008). Older people's ability to wait is reduced compared to younger people. Furthermore, there is an associated link between UI and frailty in older people (Thom et al. 1997; Thirugnanasothy 2010). Some older people accept UI as part of the ageing process, therefore do not seek help from their GP, and are not aware that treatment is available (NICE 2013c).

Diagnostic assessment in people with UI is found to be inconsistent (Wagg et al. 2007). A systematic review by Martin et al. (2006) reported that assessment, management, and care remain inconsistent, with some people being cared for by their GPs and nurses while others were referred to specialists in secondary care. Evidence suggests that continence care received by older people is often of poor quality and is dependent on the attitude of care staff (Nazarko 2008; Thirugnanasothy 2010), whose approach may be the use of continence pads instead of making a systematic continence assessment, which should include taking a detailed history, undertaking appropriate investigation, physical examination, and assessment of activities of living and medication.

Audit findings by the RCP about the services and quality of care of people with bladder and bowel incontinence in England, Wales, and Northern Ireland in 2010 provided detailed descriptions of the care given to 18,253 people with continence problems in a variety of NHS settings such as hospital wards, hospital outpatient clinics, mental health hospitals, GP surgeries, and care homes (RCP 2011). It emphasised that 'a good continence service should be led by continence specialists, with services (e.g. assessment, investigation) linked to each other so that people progress easily through the service, from assessment to successful treatment, and do not get "stuck" or "forgotten" at any stage' (RCP 2011, p. 8). Only 55% of continence services in hospital in their sample were found to be integrated. A lack of joined-up care is highlighted in an example of a person informing ward staff that they have incontinence—'they may be given pads to take home but no further information is provided, and plans for assessment and treatment of their incontinence are not made' (RCP 2011, p. 16). More worryingly, nearly one third of older patients were not given a physical examination, which is a necessary aspect of assessment. Feedback from patient groups about their user experiences also highlighted that some staff were deemed unreliable and needed training (RCP 2011). Assessment of older people with UI can be undertaken at a number of levels using different combinations of tests (NICE 2015b).

Some of the difficulties experienced by older people with UI could be minimised. Furthermore, from the perspective of carers of older people, caring for someone at home who has incontinence can pose as a stressor that could result in possible relocation to a care home (Board and Cooper 2013). It is therefore essential that health-care professionals conduct appropriate assessment and challenge their own approach and preferences in regard to containment materials, teaching, and supervision. NICE (2015b, p. 11) noted that many people with UI were not performing pelvic floor muscle exercises for 'many years with no improvement in their symptoms'. It argued that supervised pelvic floor exercise programmes with trained health-care professionals can improve symptoms significantly, thus reducing the need for invasive treatment or surgery. Pelvic floor muscle training is recommended as the first-line treatment alongside bladder training for people with mixed UI, who are able to contract their pelvic floor muscles (NICE 2015b). The Department of Health (DH) (DH 2010, p. 47) advocates the need for 'co-ordinated, consistent and accessible services [to] exist between health and social care organisations that work in partnership with other relevant agencies'.

Think about this ...

Reflect on 6 people you have cared for – how many had a comprehensive continence assessment carried out on them. If any did not think about why this might have been the case.

Review the continence services provided in your hospital and community – what sorts of services are available. Make sure you know how to access them and who are the key specialists that you can call on for advice.

Do you know how to teach pelvic floor exercises? If not find out how to and when it would be appropriate to teach them. They are useful for men and women.

In order to maintain continence older people rely on a functional urinary tract and pelvic floor, adequate cognition 'to interpret the desire to void' and find a toilet, and 'mobility and dexterity' to enable them to walk safely to the toilet (Gibson and Wagg 2014, p. 159). For older and frail people, the current gold standard 'to achieve an improvement in continence and increased spontaneous independent toileting is prompted voiding with functional incidental training' (Gibson and Wagg 2014, p. 158).

The three common types of UI management highlighted by NICE are conservative, pharmacological, or surgical (NICE 2013c). Conservative management refers to therapies such as lifestyle interventions and physical, behavioural, and non-therapeutic interventions (such as products that collect or contain leakage), while pharmacological treatment tends to include antimuscarinic drugs as well as oestrogens (NICE 2013c). Surgical or other invasive treatment may be an option when other treatments fail to treat the symptoms.

The Care Campaign was launched by the Patients Association and the Nursing Standard in 2011 to help address the four key concerns users and their families have (Buswell 2013). The CARE acronym helps to signpost nurses to (a) communicate with compassion; (b) assist with toileting, ensuring dignity; (c) relieve pain effectively; and (d) encourage adequate nutrition. A review of this campaign showcased some good examples of innovative and best practice in toileting, an example being enhanced signage to help people with visual impairment or dementia to locate the toilet with greater ease (Buswell 2013).

An approach using a trigger question such as "Do you have a bladder or bowel problem?" or "Does your bladder ever cause you embarrassment, pain or concern?" can facilitate an opportunity for the older person to share about their problem relating to incontinence and for the nurse to offer an assessment (DH 2010, p. 53). Families and carers should also be asked similar questions about the person they are providing care to.

All health-care professionals caring for older people with UI should have adequate and core competencies in the treatment of incontinence, and be able to demonstrate interprofessional working to ensure quality and dignified care. Raising the awareness of incontinence as a 'geriatric giant' is the responsibility of all health-care professionals. Patients and professionals need to stop accepting incontinence as 'an inevitable part of ageing' (Gibson and Wagg 2014, p. 160).

Key points on UI

- UI is common. About a third of women and one in seven men aged 65 or more experience UI.
- UI is under-reported.
- Using trigger questions such as "Have you a bladder or bowel problem?" is good practice. A positive response to such a trigger question should result in an offer of an initial bladder and bowel continence assessment (DH 2010, p. 53).
- The management of UI generally comprises three types: conservative, pharmacological, or surgical.
- It is recommended that people with UI complete a bladder diary for a minimum of three days and be given advice about the impact that lifestyle changes can have (NICE 2015b).
- Containment products should be offered as a temporary coping strategy, or as long-term management if treatment is unsuccessful.
- Women with stress or mixed UI who are able to contract their pelvic floor muscles are offered a trial of supervised pelvic floor muscle training of at least three months' duration as first-line treatment (NICE 2015b).
- Long-term treatment with indwelling urethral catheters should be considered only if individuals have received an assessment and discussion about the practicalities and potential complications (NICE 2015b).
- Outcomes are measured using an evidence-based tool (DH 2010, p. 13).
- Good practice should ensure that dietary and medication needs are met (and regularly reviewed) (DH 2010, p. 14).
- Nurses need to (a) communicate with compassion; (b) assist with toileting, ensuring dignity; (c) relieve pain effectively; and (d) encourage adequate nutrition.
- Faecal incontinence may accompany UI: discuss this with a specialist continence advisor/ nurse.

Pain

Like UI, experiencing pain in old age should not be seen as an aspect of normal ageing. Sadly, pain is not often managed effectively by older people; nurses seldom acknowledge or recognise this difficulty (Schofield 2013). Attempts to draw attention to this aspect of nursing care remain limited and challenging. Furthermore, pain management in older people tends to be dominated by a medical model 'that views pain as a warning sign of tissue injury or damage' (Keefe et al. 2013, p. 89). Since the launch by the British Geriatrics Society of its Pain in Older People Special Interest Group (SIG) in 2015, an editorial by the journal *Pain* on 'Is there such as thing as geriatric pain?' followed by action by the International Association for the Study of

Pain to designate 2006-7 as an International Year Against Pain in Older Persons, there is a drive to acknowledge pain and ageing as an entity in its own right (Jones and Schofield 2011). However, much more is needed to address this challenge, in particular where assessment of pain in older people are concerned (Herr 2011; Gregory 2015).

Understanding what pain is and how it affects an older person are equally important. It is widely accepted that pain is 'whatever the person experiencing pain says it is, existing whenever the person communicates or demonstrates (voluntarily or involuntarily) it does' (adapted by DH, 2010, from McCaffrey, 1968) and an unpleasant sensory and emotional experience associated with actual or potential tissue damage or described in terms of such damage (Merskey and Bogduk 1994). These definitions embrace 'both the subjective and the complex experience and include acute, chronic, intermittent, temporary, long term, acute on chronic pain and pain experienced at the end of life' (DH 2010, p. 155).

Nurses need to understand that there are similarities and differences between various types of pain, e.g. acute, chronic, cancer, and non-cancer (Jones and Schofield 2011), in order to make accurate pain assessment. Pain of less than 12 weeks' duration is considered acute while chronic pain is pain of more than 12 weeks or that persists after the expected period of healing. With acute pain, there is some association with hospital admission due to trauma, surgical intervention, or infections (Rantala et al. 2014). While its prevalence varies by gender and site of pain, 50% of older people living in the community and 80% of those living in care homes experience chronic pain (Schofield 2013, 2017). Older people may be at greater risk of inadequate pain treatment for cancer; thus, it is important that health-care professionals employ appropriate strategies to reduce under treatment for cancer pain (The British Pain Society 2010).

The most common sites of pain in older people are hip, knee, shoulder, and back (Macfarlane et al. 2005). The most frequently reported are 'osteoarthritic back pain, especially in the low back or neck (around 65%), musculoskeletal pain (around 40%), peripheral neuropathic pain (typically due to diabetes or post herpetic neuralgia, 35%), and chronic joint pain' (15%-25%) (Molton and Terrill 2014, p. 197).

The impact of pain on older people cannot be underestimated and remains an under-recognised aspect of care across all care settings (Herr 2010; Berry 2013; Gregory, 2015). Pain can impact on the quality of life (Brown 2011; Hadjistavropoulos et al. 2014). Studies by Kunz et al. (2009) and Corbett et al. (2012) found a direct correlation between severity of cognitive impairment and under-treatment of pain; the latter can result in restricted mobility, problems with gait and increase risk of falls, increase in isolation, and disturbance in sleep (Corbett et al. 2012; Gregory 2015). A person with cognitive impairment and pain can be agitated and aggressive which, in turn, are considered as challenging by health-care professionals (McAuliffe et al. 2012). This further poses a barrier to effective pain management owing to insufficient assessment and the inability of the individual to communicate about their pain (Chang et al. 2011; Rantala et al. 2014; Gregory 2015). Hence, an essential nursing approach should include not only the 'biological aspects of the experience of pain (i.e. intensity, quality and location) but also the functional and psycho-social aspects' (Jones and Schofield 2011, p. 196).

From a biological context, the existence of co-morbid conditions in older people can increase their risk of pain and make pain management challenging and complicated (Keefe et al. 2013); for example, because of age-related physiological changes that modify drug absorption, bioavailability, and transit time, pain management can be challenging (Fine 2009). The increase in pain perception threshold in older people and structural and functional changes of peripheral and central nociceptive pathways could further increase older people's risk of injury (Jones and Schofield 2011). Changes in vision, hearing, and cognition, as well as attitudes and beliefs, of health-care professionals and patients can make pain assessment challenging (Abdulla et al. 2013).

Increased pain in older people can also be caused by psychological distress such as depression, anxiety, and mood disorders (Keefe et al. 2013). From a social perspective, social isolation, and socio-economic status are two factors that have an especially important impact on pain and disability in older adults (Keefe et al. 2013). Older people often encounter significant losses, including their social status, death of a spouse and close friends, as well as their independence (Karp et al. 2008; Keefe et al. 2013). Experience of the difficulty maintaining social relationships, through greater restrictions in social and leisure activities and reduced functional abilities, can contribute to greater social isolation and exacerbation of persistent pain conditions (Gignac et al. 2008; Kharicha et al. 2017).

Assessing pain may be even more challenging in the presence of severe cognitive impairment, communication difficulties, or language and cultural barriers. Guidance from the Royal College of Physicians, British Geriatrics Society, and British Pain Society (2007, reviewed 2010) emphasises that key components of an assessment of pain should include the use of alternative words to describe pain when making a direct enquiry about the presence of pain, observing signs of pain especially among those with cognitive/communication impairment, and getting a description of the pain including the sensory and affective dimensions as well as the impact of the individual in relation to function and participation in activities.

In hospital settings, getting a pain score is considered the fifth vital sign that is included in routine vital sign observations (Gregory 2015). Getting the patient to self-report about their pain experience is deemed as a reliable and accurate approach to assessment (Hadjistavropoulos et al. 2014). There are a number of self-report pain scales available; the numerical rating scale (NRS) and verbal descriptor scale (VDS) are the two most commonly known (Gregory 2015). With the NRS, the person is asked to rate their pain on a 0–10 scale, with a score of 0 being no pain and ten, the worst pain imaginable (Gregory 2015). With the VDS, the person is required to describe the severity of pain, such as 'no pain', 'mild pain', 'moderate pain', and 'severe pain'. Some adaptation to VDS to include a numerical descriptor scale means that pain score can be documented with no pain scoring 0, mild pain with a score of 1, moderate as 2, and severe as 3 (Gregory 2015). Its ease of use is reflected in the higher percentage of users among people with dementia (90%) compared with 60% using the NRS (Bird 2005). A self-report scale such as the Pain Thermometer or a coloured Visual Analogue Scale (Scherder and Bouma 2000) is considered more appropriate for use with older people. The Brief Pain Inventory (Keller et al. 2004) is useful for multidimensional assessment in older people with minimal cognitive impairment (RCP, British Geriatrics Society and British Pain Society 2007, reviewed 2010).

Observing an older person's behaviour when undertaking a pain assessment is also key to effective pain assessment and management; this is advocated in particular for people whose communication and cognition are impaired. It is easily assumed that an individual who displays a calm appearance does not have as much pain as someone who grimaces and is tense (Gregory 2015). For observational pain assessment, the Abbey Pain Scale (Abbey et al. 2004) is found to be quick and easy to use (Royal College of Physicians, British Geriatrics Society and British Pain Society 2007, reviewed 2010). Despite its advantage in raising awareness when trialled in secondary care, its subjectivity may be considered a disadvantage (Gregory 2012).

Molton and Terrill (2014) suggest an alternative option for assessing pain through the use of proxy-rating or non-verbal behavioural indicator pain assessment scales (Herr et al. 2006), which rely on caregivers or health-care professionals to note any physiological and behavioural changes that might signal the presence or severity of or a change in pain. Hence, it is imperative to assess a person's cognitive status to decide which assessment tool is appropriate, whether one or more tools are utilised to ensure accuracy (Corbett et al. 2012).

Some interventions may be appropriate for older people. Psychological interventions, such as cognitive behavioural therapy (CBT), may be effective in reducing chronic pain and improving disability and mood in adults. Studies that focused on older people are limited where small samples were involved, making it difficult to generalise (Schofield 2013). However, there is some evidence to support the use of CBT in nursing homes (Keefe et al. 2013; Schofield 2013).

Pharmacological interventions tend to aim at changing sensory transmission to the cerebral cortex (Jett 2014). The use of non-narcotic analgesics in the relief of physical pain in older people may be effective although non-steroidal anti-inflammatory drug usage is known to be associated with gastrointestinal bleeding and renal dysfunction (Cooper and Burfield 2010). Nurses need to be aware and anticipate a number of adverse outcomes and differences in sensitivities and toxicities arising from medications such as opiates and the worry of older people in becoming 'addicted' (Molton and Terrill 2014).

Pain can present as a risk factor for falls in older people (Schofield 2017). Generally, activities that focus on strengthening, flexibility, and endurance are tailored to the functional ability of older people to help them increase their physical activities which in turn can help reduce their pain are advocated (Schofield 2013). Bearing in mind that older people who have severe, persistent pain are twice as likely to experience sleep difficulties (Chen et al. 2011), with more than 40% of middle-aged and older people suffering from chronic sleep deprivation (Artner et al. 2013), it is equally important that nurses recognise the impact of pain on sleep in older people and their daily activities (see Audrey's story in Appendix 1).

Needless to say, pain in older people is under assessed (Molton and Terrill 2014; Gregory 2015). With more education and training, nurses and other health-care professionals can become more equipped to be effective in their assessment, planning, and implementing responsive and person-centred care of older people experiencing pain, be it acute, chronic, and persistent. The ultimate goals of pain management in older people should include the promotion of comfort, maintaining functional and self-care where possible, and making choice and balancing risk and benefits of treatment and care options (Jett 2014).

Key points on pain

- Pain in older people, across settings, remains under-assessed.
- There are similarities and differences between various types of pain, e.g. acute, chronic, cancer, and non-cancer (Jones and Schofield 2011).
- Helping older people to manage pain can be challenging; nurses should explore the biological aspects of the experience of pain (i.e. intensity, quality, and location) as well as the functional and psychosocial aspects.
- Various tools are available to assess pain in older people, depending on the presence of cognitive/communication impairment.

Difficulty with mobility and physical activity

General health and well-being in later life can make a difference to the quality of life experienced by older people (Age UK 2017). Not surprisingly, being active regularly has physical, psychological, and social benefits (Eliopoulos 2014). However, with age, it becomes more challenging to maintain a physically active status, compounded by the presence of co-morbidity and for some, chronic health problems such as osteoporosis, obesity, joint stiffness, or immobility (Eliopoulos 2014). Ageing not only leads to a decline in functional capacity but also affects the person's strength, balance, bone density, and flexibility by about 10% each decade (British Heart Foundation, BHF 2012). This gradual loss in physical function can impact on the person's independence as they age. Consequently, some older people experience difficulty with mobility. Age UK (2017) stated that '18% of adults aged 60-69 have a mobility difficulty, and 38% of adults aged 70+ do'. Being aware of the various factors that might limit an older person's mobility and the level of activity adequate to maintain their health as well as improve mobility would help nurses and other health-care professionals in motivating older persons in regaining their strength and stamina. This in turn, can help enhance the quality of life in older people (Nelson et al. 2007). Sedentary behaviour is ranked among the ten leading causes of death worldwide by the World Health Organization (British Heart Foundation 2017).

According to Age UK (2015), people aged 75 years or more are less likely to meet the minimum levels of physical activity necessary to attain health benefits. In England alone, only 19% of those aged 65-74 reported meeting this minimum level. Worryingly, about 40% of adults aged 50 years or more are 'completely inactive' (Skelton et al. 2011, p. 122).

Older people may have difficulty in understanding the difference between physical activity and exercise. As nurses, knowing this difference can help older people understand what things do to improve their health without undue risk. Physical activity, being any activity that 'uses the muscular system in some exertion' (such as gardening, walking, or housework), is also associated with better cognitive functioning, reduction in disability, improvement in sleep as well as reduction of risks in some conditions such as cardiovascular, osteoporosis, obesity, and diabetes in old age (Skelton et al. 2011, p. 123). Active living such as walking at least 6 miles a week can reduce the risk of developing memory problems by half (Erickson et al. 2010). In women aged 65-74, weekly strength training exercise is found to improve their cognitive ability (Davis et al. 2010). Exercise is a term that refers to 'any structured activity that is aimed at improving one or more components of fitness (strength, endurance, balance, flexibility, etc.)' (Skelton et al. 2011, p. 123).

By contrast, being immobile for a few weeks can have detrimental effect on the person's muscle strength, mass, and power (Skelton et al. 2011). In hospital settings, bed rest in older people is known to lead to adverse impact such as cardiac deconditioning, decreased lung function, loss of muscle mass, strength, and endurance as well as skin integrity (Nigam et al. 2009). In settings such as care homes, residents are known to spend extended periods of inactivity (sitting or lying down) which could result in a reduction of bone mineral loss (immobility). Having adequate sleep and activity can enhance physical, emotional, and cognitive functioning while poor sleep and reduced functional capacity can compromise the individual's capacity for independence and well-being (Touhy and Jett 2014).

Much can be done by nurses to promote activity and movement in older people whilst recognising their difficulty in mobility. In frail older people, evidence suggests that promoting circulation through physical activity and movement can reduce the undesirable complications of immobility and sedentary lifestyle including gravitational oedema, limb contractures, pressure sores as well as constipation (BHFNC 2011; BHF 2012).

The NHS recommends minimum levels of exercise by healthy older people (NHS Choices 2014). Older people should aim to be active every day with a weekly target of 150 minutes, in bouts of ten minutes or more (NHS Choices 2014; Public Health England 2016). However, this may not be realistic or safe for older people in hospitals, residential care homes, or nursing homes even though care staff have to ensure that older patients can stand and mobilise as early as possible after illnesses (Oliver et al. 2014). Older people should aim to be active daily and to reduce the time they spend sitting still and ideally have about up to two-and-a half hours per week of moderate intensity activity (in bouts of ten minutes or more) (Age UK 2017). For those at risk of falls, it is recommended that they should 'incorporate physical activity to improve balance and coordination on at least two days a week' (British Heart Foundation 2015, p. 14). Other activities that improve their muscle strength and improve their balance and coordination are to be encouraged (Skelton et al. 2011) since being mobile and physically active can be particularly beneficial such as in the prevention for loneliness (Victor et al. 2005) particularly if this involves group activities.

Assessment of mobility in older people needs to take into account factors such as their gait and balance. In hospital settings, the use of the Elderly Mobility Scale (EMS) (Smith 1994) helps health-care professionals to assess seven functional activities including bed mobility, transfers, and bodily reaction to perturbation (Chiu et al. 2003). As a validated tool for use in hospital settings, the EMS takes into account locomotion, balance, and key changes in position which can help to identify someone at risk of falling (Spilg et al. 2003). Its use to provide mobility profiles for people in residential care settings has helped Yu et al. (2007) in allocating individuals to appropriate care settings. Although normally used by physiotherapists in mobility assessment, its ease of use and need for minimal training should make it easily accessible for nurses to have a better understanding of mobility and its key components for assessment.

In primary care, practitioners can use a validated screening tool such as the General Practice Physical Activity Questionnaire (GPPAQ) to assess the physical activity levels of adults (16-74 years). This tool provides a simple four-level physical activity index (PAI) which can assist practitioners in deciding when to offer interventions to increase physical activity (Department of Health, England, 2013). Nurses also need to consider other factors such as good nutrition to prevent and manage musculoskeletal problems and a balanced diet to help maintain bone health in older people under their care.

Key points in mobility and physical activity

- General health and well-being in later life can make a difference to the quality of life.
- The NHS recommends minimum levels of exercise for healthy older people.
- Older people should aim to be active every day with a weekly target of 150 minutes, in bouts of ten minutes or more.
- Using tools such as EMS or GPPAQ can help provide health-care professionals with a mobility profile of the individual in their care.
- Interprofessional working is key to help maintain and develop a programme to maintain or increase the person's mobility.

Loneliness

Loneliness among older people is increasingly recognised as a public health problem (Kharicha et al. 2017). Importantly, other experiences associated with ageing, such as loss (e.g. family and friends), declining health and financial status, restricted mobility, and changes in relationships within the family and communities are all linked closely to loneliness (Bernard 2013; Nicolaisen and Thorsen 2014; Age UK 2017). In England alone, 51% of all people over 75 live alone and 5 million older people say the television is their main form of company (NHS Choices 2014). 12.04% or 1.2 million older people (65 and over in England) are said to be persistently/chronically lonely (Marmot et al. 2016). Having reduced social contact, being alone, isolation, and feelings of loneliness are found to be associated with reduced quality of old people's lives (Victor 2011); this adversely affects their health, increases their risk of premature death by about 25% (Holt-Lunstad et al. 2015), and leads to increased use of health- and social-care services (Windle et al. 2011). Hence, it is important that health-care professionals are aware of this issue and the factors associated with it, its potential impact and be alert to this risk when working with this group of the population.

The terms loneliness, social isolation, and living alone are used interchangeably in the literature, although they are three distinct linked concepts (Jack 2013). Living alone–living on your own without others–is the simplest and most objective term to measure (Jack 2013). Loneliness tends to be categorised as a subjective negative feeling i.e. how individuals feel about their level and quality of social contact and engagement while social isolation is 'an objective state mediated by the presence or absence of strong social networks' (Collins 2014, p. 3). Importantly, although a person can have extensive connections he/she can still experience the subjective feeling of loneliness. Likewise, he/she can be objectively isolated but not experience associated negative emotions (Collins 2014). Some literature refers to emotional and social loneliness. 'Emotional loneliness is the absence of a significant other with whom a close emotional attachment is formed (e.g. a partner or best friend) and social loneliness is the absence of a social network consisting of a wide or broad group of friends, neighbours and colleagues' (Age UK Oxfordshire 2015, p. 10).

Although the mechanisms on how social isolation and loneliness affect health are not clearly understood (Courtin and Knapp 2015), a knowledge of factors that might contribute to loneliness in older people would help health-care professionals identify those at risk. Wethington and Pillemer (2014) identified the following factors that contribute to social isolation and loneliness: role loss, living alone, bereavement, health changes, or deterioration and poverty as well as the ageing of baby boomers who have lower rates of marriage, higher levels of divorce, and fewer children (Hawkley et al. 2010). For example, having to give up driving could restrict older people's opportunities to maintain social interaction outside the home. A reduced income can also result in older people restricting their leisure and social activities and travelling. Emerging changes such as altered mobility, cognitive impairment, hearing/sight changes, or incontinence could lead to a change in lifestyles that could have less meaningful engagement with others (Nicholson 2012).

The impact of loneliness on health needs to be recognised by health-care professionals; this can be 'as harmful to health as smoking 15 cigarettes a day, and is more damaging than obesity' (Holt-Lunstad et al. 2010). Not only are lonely individuals at a higher risk of the onset of disability, they are also at greater risk of cognitive decline (Victor 2011). Evidence also suggests that being lonely can have an impact on an individual's BP, with those being lonely having higher BP than their less lonely peers (Windle et al. 2011). A five-year analysis in middle-aged and older people by Hawkley et al. (2010) found loneliness to be a predictive factor of increased systolic BP independent of, e.g., age, gender, race, cardiovascular risk factors, medications, health conditions, and the effects of depressive symptoms. Loneliness is also associated with depression and higher rates of mortality (Pitkala et al. 2009). Furthermore, 'widowhood, housing tenure, and poor self-reported health are associated with higher prevalence of loneliness while household size is inversely associated' (Iparraguirre 2016, p. 15).

Little is known about what nurses do to address loneliness in older people even though they are among the few people with whom lonely older people have ongoing contact (Jopling 2015). Thus, nurses and other health-care professionals need to be mindful of the stigma attached to loneliness that can potentially limit older people to seek help or willingly voice their needs (Griffin 2010). There may be the assumption that loneliness is a social rather than health problem and is best dealt with by social services and other organisations such as charities. Much more can be done in nurse education to broaden the curriculum to ensure that nurses are taught now to recognise signs of loneliness (not necessary in older people but other age groups such as young adults) and to make appropriate referrals and impart information about the types of services available to support and maintain existing relationships that older people have already as well as supporting them to develop new relationships. Increasingly nurses are being involved in social prescribing which can be used to address loneliness for some people (see Chapter 5). Furthermore, communication skills to ensure that nurses are confident about using 'guided conversation' and motivational interviewing (see Chapter 4) are important to develop. It is also worthwhile to recognise that 'when individuals feel lonely, they think and act differently than when they do not feel lonely' (Masi et al. 2011, p. 222).

Other factors need to be considered. For example, the use of technology such as the internet may not be easily accessible and appealing to older people (Jopling 2015). Having good infrastructure such as transport is essential to help older people maintain their social 'connections' (Jopling 2015), even though its provision and maintenance will have cost implications in the community.

The use of psychological interventions, for example, the use of CBT have gained increased prominence. Mindfulness and CBT are recommended for use among people with depression (NICE Clinical Guidance 90 2009). The premise of CBT intervention is to teach lonely individuals to identify negative thoughts automatically (Masi et al. 2011, p. 223). However, its use as an intervention for loneliness is not widely offered by organisations to combat loneliness despite a meta-analysis of interventions to reduce loneliness by Masi et al. (2011, p. 259) indicating that 'correcting maladaptive social cognition offers the best chance for reducing loneliness'.

Through a therapeutic relationship, nurses are ideally placed to assess whether older people in their care are at risk of being socially isolated and determine if they feel lonely or not. There is recognition that apart from preventative approaches to loneliness, an asset-based (or strengths-based) approach could offer an alternative by rejecting the focus on the needs of older people but rather, on the potential of the individual, their skills and expertise, relationships as well as community resources (Jopling 2015). Typically, those adopting this approach would go some way to informing, empowering, and connecting people (Jopling 2015). In practice, the nurse could be familiar with updated information about services/networks for older people, recognise the specific skills that older people have, and empower them to maintain independence.

Key points on loneliness

- Loneliness and isolation are common problems amongst older people and can have a profound impact on their health and well-being.
- Nurses are ideally placed to assess whether older people in their care are at risk of being socially isolated and determine if they feel lonely or not. They are also able to recommend (or prescribe) ways to overcome loneliness.
- A wide range of biological, psychological, and social factors contribute to loneliness in older people and these include physical and mental health of individuals, restricted mobility and limited transport, and social interactions.

Summary of key messages

- Understanding the common difficulties encountered by older people will assist nurses and other health- and social-care professionals to be attuned to their complexity.
- Many difficulties that older people experience are interlinked and can be challenging to address. Careful assessment, underpinned by sensitive communication and accurate measurement, is critical to their management.
- Nurses need to be active and equal members of multidisciplinary teams in order to ensure that older people receive the best possible care based on every relevant source of knowledge and skill at their disposal.

References

Abbey, Jennifer, Neil Piller, Anita De Bellis, Adrian Esterman, Deborah Parker, Lynne Giles and Belinda Lowcay. 2004. "The Abbey pain scale: A 1-minute numerical indicator for people with end-stage dementia." *International Journal of Palliative Nursing* 10, 6–13.
Abdulla, Aza, Adams Nicola, Bone Margaret, Elliott Alison M, Gaffin Jean, Jones Derek, Knaggs Roger, Martin Denis, Sampson Lisa, Schofield Pat and British Geriatric Society. 2013. "Guidance on the management of pain in older people." *Age and Ageing* 42, Suppl 1, i1–i57.
Age UK Oxfordshire. 2011. *Safeguarding the convoy: A call to action from the campaign to end loneliness.* Oxford: Age UK Oxfordshire.
Age UK. 2015. Later life in the United Kingdom. August.
Age UK. 2017. Later life in the United Kingdom. August. www.ageuk.org.uk/Documents/EN-GB/Fact sheets/Later_Life_UK_factsheet.pdf?dtrk=true
Artner, Juraj, Balkan Cakir, Jane-Anna Spiekermann, Stephan Kurz, Frank Leucht, Heiko Reichel and Friederike Lettig. 2013. "Prevalence of sleep deprivation in patients with chronic neck and back pain: A retrospective evaluation of 1016 patients." *Journal of Pain Research* 6, 1–6.
Bernard, Sylvia. 2013. "Loneliness and social isolation among older people in North Yorkshire." Working Paper No. WP 2565. Social Policy Research Unit, University of York, York.
Berry, Lisa. 2013 "Controlling patients' pain. Editorial." *Nursing Older People* 25, 7, 5.
Bird, Joanna. 2005 "Assessing pain in older people." *Nursing Standard* 19, 19, 45–52.
Board, Michele and Karen Cooper. 2013. Chapter 5. "Physical aspects of ageing." In: *Caring for older people in nursing*, edited by Sue Barker, 79–102. London: Sage.
British Geriatrics Society. 2016a. "Assessment and management of falls." www.bgs.org.uk/falls-assessment-management/cga-toolkit-category/assessment-and-management-of-falls (Accessed 25 October 2017).
British Geriatrics Society. 2016b. "Urinary incontinence." www.bgs.org.uk/urinary-incontinence/cga-toolkit-category/how-cga/cga-assessment/cga-specific-conditions/cga-urinary-incontinence/cga-med-con-incontinence.
British Heart Foundation National Centre (BHFNC) for Physical Activity and Health, Loughborough University. 2011. Physical activities for older adults (65+ years).
British Heart Foundation. 2012. Evidence briefing. Physical activity for older adults (65+ years). Loughborough University: BHF National Centre Physical Activity+Health.
British Heart Foundation. 2015. "Physical activities statistics 2015." www.bhf.org.uk/~/media/files/.../bhf_physical-activity-statistics-2015_new.pdf
British Heart Foundation. 2017. Physical inactivity and sedentary behaviour report. British Heart Foundation.
Brown, Donna. 2011. "Pain assessment with cognitively impaired older people in the acute hospital setting." *British Journal of Pain* 5, 3, 18–22.
Buswell, Jane. 2013. "What guidance and resources are available to help nurses ensure they meet the privacy and dignity needs of older adults in terms of continence?" www.bgs.org.uk/index.php/practicequestions/2499-qa-dignity-continence (Accessed 10 October 2015).
Chang, Sung Ok, Younjae Oh, Eun Young Park, Geun Myun Kim and Suk Yong Kil E. 2011. "Concept analysis of nurses' identification of pain in demented patients in a nursing home: Development of a hybrid model." *Pain Management Nursing* 12, 2, 61–69.
Chen, Qian, Laura L. Hayman, Robert G. Shmerling and Simon G. Leveille. 2011. "Characteristics of persistent pain associated with sleep difficulty in older adults: The maintenance of balance, independent living, intellect, and zest in the elderly (MOBILIZE) Boston study." *Journal of the American Geriatrics Society* 59, 1385–1392.
Chiu, Arlene Y.Y., Stephanie S.Y. Au-Yeung and Simon K. Lo. 2003. "A comparison of four functional tests in discriminating fallers from non-fallers in older people." *Disability and Rehabilitation* 25, 45–50.
Collins, Emma. 2014. "Preventing social isolation and loneliness in older people. Evidence summaries to support social services in Scotland." The Institute for Research and Innovation in Social Services (IRISS). www.scotland.gov.uk/about/performance/scotperforms/outcome/pubserv
Cooper, James W., and Allison H. Burfield. 2010. "Assessment and management of chronic pain in the older adult." *Journal of the American Pharmacists Association* 50, e89–e102.
Corbett, Anne, Bettina Husebo, Marzia Malcangio, Amelia Staniland, Jiska Cohen-Mansfield, Dag Aarsland and Clive Ballard. 2012. "Assessment and treatment of pain in people with dementia." *Nature Reviews Neurology* 8, 5, 264–274.

Cornwell, Jocelyn, Ross Levenson, Lara Sonola and Emmi Poteliakhoff. 2012. *Continuity of care for older hospital patients: A call for action*. London: The King's Fund. www.kingsfund.org.uk/publications/continuity-care-older-hospital-patients (Accessed 10 July 2015).

Courtin, Emilie and Martin Knapp. 2015. "Social isolation, loneliness and health in old age: A scoping review." *Health and Social Care in the Community* 25, 3, 799–812. doi: 10.1111/hsc.12311.

Davis, Jennifer, Carlo Marra, Lynn Beattie, Clare Robertson, Mehdi Najafzadeh, Peter Graf, Lindsay S. Nagamatsu and Teresa Liu-Ambrose. 2010. "Sustained cognitive and economic benefits of resistance training among community-dwelling senior women: A 1-year follow-up study of the brain power study." *Archives of Internal Medicine* 170, 22, 2036–2038.

Department of Health. 2010. *How to use Essence of Care 2010. Benchmarks for fundamental aspects of care*. England: Department of Health, England.

Department of Health. 2012. "Improving outcomes and supporting transparency" as cited on NHS Choices website. www.nhs.uk/Scorecard/Pages/IndicatorFacts.aspx?MetricId=8135

Department of Health. 2013. General practice physical activity questionnaire. www.gov.uk/government/publications/general-practice-physical-activity-questionnaire-gppaq (Accessed 25 October 2017).

Dollard, Joanne, Annette Braunack-Meyer, Khim Horton and Simon Vanlint. 2014. "Why older women do or do not seek help from GP after a fall: A qualitative study." *Family Practice* 31, 2, 222–228.

Eliopoulos, Charlotte. 2014. *Gerontological nursing*. Eighth Edition. Philadelphia: Wolters Kluwer/Lippincott Williams & Wilkins.

Erickson, Kirk I., Cyrus A. Raji, Oscar L. Lopez, James T. Becker, C. Rosana, A.B. Newman, H.M. Gach, Paul Thompson, April J. Ho and Lewis H. Kuller. 2010. "Physical activity predicts gray matter volume in late adulthood: The Cardiovascular Health Study." *Neurology* 75, 1415–1422.

Fenton, Kevin. 2017. "A new focus on Falls Prevention." Public Health England. https://publichealthmatters.blog.gov.uk/2017/01/25/a-new-focus-on-falls-prevention/ (Accessed 25 October 2017).

Fine, Perry G. 2009. "Chronic pain management in older adults: Special considerations." *Journal of Pain and Symptom Management* 38, S4–14.

Foundation Trust Network. 2012. *FTN benchmarking: Driving improvement in elderly care services*. London: Foundation Trust Network. www.nhsproviders.org/resource-library/ftnbenchmarking-elderly-care-services-briefing-2012/ (Accessed 10 July 2015).

Gibson, William and Adrian Wagg. 2014. "New horizons: Urinary incontinence in older people." *Age and Ageing* 43, 157–163.

Gignac, Monique AM., Catherine L. Backman, Aileen M. Davis, Diane Lacaille, Cristian A Mattison, Pamela Montie and Elizabeth M. Badley. 2008. "Understanding social role participation: What matters to people with arthritis?" *The Journal of Rheumatology* 35, 1655–1663.

Gregory, Julie. 2012. "How to assess pain in people who have difficulty communicating? A practice development project identifying a pain assessment tool for acute care." *International Practice Development Journal* 2, 2, 1–22.

Gregory, Julie. 2015. "The complexity of pain assessment in older people." *Nursing Older People* 27, 8, 16–21.

Griffin, Jo. 2010. The lonely society? London: Mental Health Foundation. www.mentalhealth.org.uk/content/assets/PDF/publications/the_lonely_society_report.pdf?view=Standard (Accessed 18 August 2015).

Hadjistavropoulos, Thomas, Keela Herr, Kenneth Prkachin, Kenneth Craig, Stephen Gibson, Albert Lukas and Jonathan Smith. 2014. "Pain assessment in elderly adults with dementia." *The Lancet. Neurology* 13, 12, 1216–1227.

Hawkley, Louise C., Ronald A. Thisted and John T. Cacioppo. 2010. "Loneliness predicts increased blood pressure: 5-year cross-lagged analyses in middle-aged and older adults." *Psychology and Aging* 25, 1, 132–141.

Health and Social Care Information Centre (HSCIC). 2014. Focus on The Health and Care of Older People. London: HSCIC. https://files.digital.nhs.uk/publicationimport/pub14xxx/pub14369/focu-on-hac-op-main-pub-doc%201.1.pdf (Accessed 5th June 2019).

Health Survey for England. 2015. "Health, social care and lifestyles. Summary of key findings." National Statistics Publication. http://healthsurvey.hscic.gov.uk/media/37741/hse2015-summary.pdf (Accessed 23 October 2017).

Herr, Keela A. 2010. "Pain in older adults: An imperative across all health care settings." *Pain Management Nursing* 11, 2 Suppl, S1–S10.

Herr, Keela A. 2011. "Pain assessment strategies in older patients." *The Journal of Pain* 12, 3 Suppl 1, S3–S13.

Herr, Keela A., Karen Bjoro and Sheila Decker. 2006. "Tools for assessment of pain in nonverbal older adults with dementia: A state-of-the-science review." *Journal of Pain and Symptom Management* 31, 2, 170–192.

Holt-Lunstad, Julianne, Timothy B. Smith and J. Bradley Layton. 2010. "Social relationships and mortality risk: A meta-analytic review." *PLoS Med* 7, 7, e1316. https://scholarsarchive.byu.edu/cgi/viewcontent. cgi?referer=http://www.google.co.uk/url?sa=t&rct=j&q=&esrc=s&source=web&cd=2&ved=0ahUKE wisOerEuPPYAhWkBcAKHS8RAvQQFgg7MAE&url=http%3A%2F%2Fscholarsarchive.byu.edu%2F cgi%2Fviewcontent.cgi%3Farticle%3D1093%26context%3Dfacpub&usg=AOvVaw2vyFKc- j9mUHCqB9rOymwf3&httpsredir=1&article=1093&context=facpub (Accessed 20 January 2018).

Holt-Lunstad, Julianne, Timothy B. Smith, Mark Baker, Tyler Harris and David Stephenson. 2015. "Lone- liness and social isolation as risk factors for mortality: A meta-analytic review." *Perspectives on Psy- chological Science* 10, 2, 227–237. doi: 10.1177/1745691614568352.

Imison, Candace, Emmi Poteliakhoff and James Thompson. 2012. *Older people and emergency bed use: Exploring variation*. London: The King's Fund. www.kingsfund.org.uk/publications/older-people and-emergency-bed-use (Accessed 10 July 2015).

Iparraguirre, Jose. 2016. *Predicting the prevalence of loneliness at older ages*. London: Age UK.

Jack, Eleanor. 2013. Chapter 9. "Social isolation and loneliness in later life". In: *Caring for older people in nursing*, edited by Sue Barker, 165–190. London: Sage.

Jett, Kathleen F. 2014. Chapter 15. "Pain and comfort." In: *Ebersole and Hess' Gerontological Nursing and Health Aging*, Fourth Edition, edited by Theris A. Touhy and Kathleen F. Jett, 233–245. St Louis: Elsevier.

Jones, Derek and Pat Schofield. 2011. Chapter 12. "Pain and older people". In: *Evidence Informed Nursing with Older People*, edited by Debbie Tolson, Joanne Booth and Irene Schofield, 188–207. Chichester: Wiley-Blackwell.

Jopling, Kate. 2015. "Promising approaches to reducing loneliness and isolation in later life." Age UK and the Campaign to End Loneliness. https://s3-eu-central-1.amazonaws.com/content.gulbenkian. pt/wp-content/uploads/sites/18/2015/01/01175326/25-06-15-Promising-approaches-to-reducing- loneliness-and-isolation-in-later-life.pdf

Karp, Jordan F., Joseph W. Shega, Natalia E. Morone and Debra K. Weiner. 2008. "Advances in under- standing the mechanisms and management of persistent pain in older adults." *British Journal of Anaesthesia* 101: 111–20.

Keefe, Francis J., Laura Porter, Tamara Somers, Rebecca Shelby and Anava V. Wren. 2013. "Psychosocial interventions for managing pain in older adults: Outcomes and clinical implications." *British Journal of Anaesthesia* 111, 1, 89–94.

Keller, San, Carla M. Bann, Stephen L Dodd, Jeff Schein, Tito R. Mendoza TR and Charles S. Cleeland. 2004. "Validity of the brief pain inventory for use in documenting the outcomes of patients with non- cancer pain." *The Clinical Journal of Pain* 20, 309–318.

Kharicha, Kalpa, Steve Iliffe, Jill Manthorpe, Carolyn A. Chew-Graham, Mima Cattan, Claire Goodman, Maggie Kirby-Barr, Janet H. Whitehouse and Kate Walters. 2017. "What do older people experiencing loneliness think about primary care or community based interventions to reduce loneliness? A quali- tative study in England." *Health and Social Care in the Community* 25, 6, 1733–1742.

Kunz, Miriam, Veit Mylius, Siegfried Scharmann, Karsten Schepelman and Stefan Lautenbacher. 2009. "Influence of dementia on multiple components of pain." *European Journal of Pain* 13, 3, 317–325.

Macfarlane, Gary J., Gareth T. Jones and John McBeth. 2005. "Epidemiology of pain." In: *Wall and Melzack's textbook of pain*, edited by Stephen McMahon and Martin Koltzenburg, 1199–1214. Edinburgh: Churchill Livingstone.

Marmot, Michael, Zoe Oldfield, Sam Clemens, Margaret Blake, A. Phelps, James Nazroo, Andrew Steptoe, Nina Rogers, James Banks and Anni Oskala. 2016. English Longitudinal Study of Ageing: Waves 0-7, 1998-2015. [data collection]. Twenty-fifth Edition. UK Data Service. SN: 5050. doi: 10.5255/ UKDA-SN-5050-12. Figures extrapolated to national population using latest ONS Populations Estimates.

Martin, Jose Louis, Kate S. Williams, Keith R. Abrams, David A. Turner, Andrew J. Sutton, Christorpher Chapple, Phil Assassa, Christine Shaw and Francine Cheater. 2006. "Systematic review and evaluation of methods of assessing urinary incontinence." *Health Technology Assessment* 10, 6, 1–132.

Masi, Christopher, His-Yuan Chen, Louise Hawkley and John T. Cacioppo. 2011. "A meta-analysis of interventions to reduce loneliness." *Personality and Social Psychology Review* 15, 3, 219–266.

McAuliffe, Linda, Donna Brown and Deidre Fetherstonhaugh. 2012. Pain and dementia: An overview of the literature. *International Journal of Older People Nursing* 7, 3, 219–226.

Merskey, Harold and Nikolai Bogduk (eds.). 1994. Classification of chronic pain. Second Edited, International Association for the Study of Pain Task Force on Taxonomy. Seattle: ISAP Press.

Molton, Ivan R. and Alexandra L. Terrill. 2014. "Overview of persistent pain in older adults." *American Psychologist* 69, 2, 197–207.

National Health Services (NHS) Choices. 2014. "Physical activity guidelines for older adults." www.nhs.uk/livewell/fitness/pages/physical-activity-guidelines-for-adults.aspx (Accessed 10 October 2015).

National Health Services (NHS) Improvement. 2017. "The incidence and costs of inpatient falls in hospitals." London: NHSI. https://improvement.nhs.uk/resources/incidence-and-costs-inpatient-falls-hospitals/.

National Institute for Health and Care Excellence. 2009. "Depression in adults: Recognition and management. Clinical guideline 90." Manchester: National Institute for Health and Care Excellence.

National Institute for Health and Care Excellence. 2013a. "Older patients at high risk of hospital falls." Press release. NICE website. www.nice.org.uk/news/article/older-patients-at-high-risk-ofhospital-falls (Accessed 14 July 2015).

National Institute for Health and Care Excellence. 2013b. "Falls: Assessment and prevention of falls in older people." NICE Clinical Guideline 161. Manchester: National Institute for Health and Care Excellence.

National Institute for Health and Care Excellence. 2013c. "Urinary incontinence: The management of urinary incontinence in women." NICE clinical guideline 171, September.

National Institute for Health and Care Excellence. 2015a. "Falls in older people: Assessment after a fall and preventing further falls. NICE quality standard 86." London: NICE. www.nice.org.uk/ guidance/qs86 (Accessed 11 July 2015).

National Institute for Health and Care Excellence. 2015b. "Urinary incontinence in women. NICE quality standard QS 77". https://www.nice.org.uk/guidance/qs77

Nazarko, Linda. 2008. "A guide to continence assessment for community nurses." *British Journal of Community Nursing* 13, 5, 219–226.

Nelson, Miriam E., W. Jack Rejeski, Steven N. Blair, Pamela W. Duncan, James O. Judge, Abby C. King, Carol A. Macera and Carmen Castaneda-Sceppa. 2007. "Physical activity and public health in older adults: Recommendations from the American College of Sports Medicine and the American Heart Association." *Medicine and Science in Sports and Exercise* 39, 1435–1445.

Nicholson, Nicholas. 2012. "A review of social isolation: An important but underassessed condition in older adults." *Journal of Primary prevention* 33, 137–152.

Nicolaisen, Magnhild and Kirsten Thorsen. 2014. "Loneliness among men and women – a five-year follow-up study." *Aging and Mental Health* 18, 2, 194–206.

Nigam, Yamni, John Knight and Aled Jones. 2009. "Effects of bedrest 3: Musculoskeletal and immune systems, skin and self-perception." *Nursing Times* 105, 23, 16–20.

Oliver, David, Catherine Foot and Richard Humphries. 2014. *Making our health and care systems fit for an ageing population*. London: The King's Fund.

O'Riordan, Shelagh, Vasilakis Naomi, Hussain Labib, Schoo Rebecca, Whitney Julie, Windsor Julie, Horton Khim and Martin Finbarr. 2017. "Measurement of lying and standing blood pressure in hospital." *Nursing Older People* 29, 8, 20–26. doi: 10.7748/nop.2017.e961.

Pitkala, Kaisu, Routasalo Pirkko, Kautiainen, Hannu and Tilvis Reijo S. 2009. "Effects of pyschosocial group rehabiliation on health, use of health care services, and mortality of older persons suffering from loneliness: a randomised, controlled trial." *Journal of Gerontolgy: Medical Sciences* 64, 7, 792–800.

Poteliakhoff, Emmi and James Thompson. 2011. *Emergency bed use: What the numbers tell us*. London: The King's Fund. www.kingsfund.org.uk/publications/data-briefing-emergency-bed-use (Accessed 13 July 2015).

Public Health England. 2016. "Health matters- getting adult active every day." www.gov.uk/government/publications/health-matters-getting-every-adult-active-every-day. (Accessed 26 October 2017).

Ramaswamy, Bhanu and Diana Jones. 2012. Chapter 7. "Mobility." In: *Nursing Older Adults*, edited by Jan Reed, Charlotte Clarke and Ann Macfarlane, 91–109. Maidenhead: Open University Press and McGraw-Hill.

Rantala, Maija, Paivi Kankkunen P., Tarja Kvistand and Samuel Hartikainen. 2014. "Barriers to postoperative pain management in hip fracture patients with dementia as evaluated by nursing staff." *Pain Management Nursing* 15, 1, 208–219.

Royal College of Physicians. 2011. "Keeping control. What you should expect from your NHS bladder and bowel service. Based on findings from the national audit of continence care 2010." www.rcplondon.ac.uk/sites/default/files/keeping-control-2011.pdf (Accessed 12 August 2015).

Royal College of Physicians. 2012. "Report of the 2011 inpatient falls pilot audit." London: RCP. www.rcplondon.ac.uk/projects/national-audit-falls-and-bone-health-older-people

Royal College of Physicians. 2014a. "FFFAP: Report into the feasibility of a national audit of falls prevention in acute hospitals." London: RCP.

Royal College of Physicians. 2014b. "National hip fracture database annual report 2014." London: RCP.

Royal College of Physicians. 2015. "National audit of inpatient falls: Audit report 2015." London: RCP.

Royal College of Physicians. 2017. "National audit of inpatient falls Audit report 2017." www.rcplondon.ac.uk/projects/outputs/naif-audit-report-2017.

Royal College of Physicians, British Geriatrics Society and British Pain Society. 2007. "The assessment of pain in older people: National guidelines." Concise guidance to good practice series, No 8. London: RCP.

Saxer, Susi, Halfens Ruud J., de Bie Rob A. and Dassen Theo. 2008. "Prevalence and incidence of urinary incontinence of Swiss nursing home residents at admission and after six, 12 and 24 months." *Journal of Clinical Nursing* 17, 18, 2490–2496.

Scheffer, Alice C., Marieke J. Schuurmans, Nynkevan van Dijk, Truus van der Hooft and Sophia E. Rooij. 2008. "Fear of falling: Measurement strategy, prevalence, risk factors and consequences among older persons." *Age Ageing* 37, 19–24.

Scherder, Erik J.A. and Anke Bouma. 2000. "Visual analogue scales for pain assessment in Alzheimer's disease." *Gerontology* 46, 47–53.

Schofield, Patricia. 2013. "Managing chronic pain in older people." *Nursing Times* 109, 30, 26–27.

Schofield, Patricia. 2017. "Pain management in older adults." *Medicine* 45, 1, 41–45.

Skelton, Dawn, Marie McAloon and Lyle Gray. 2011. Chapter 8. "Promoting physical activity with older people." In: *Evidence informed nursing with older people*, edited by Debbie Tolson, Joanne Booth and Irene Schofield, 1121–136. Chichester: Wiley-Blackwell.

Smith, Rachael. 1994 "Validation and reliability of the elderly mobility scale." *Physiotherapy* 80, 744–747.

Snooks, Helen, Wai Yee Cheung, Stella May Gwini, Ioan Humphreys, Antonio Sánchez and Niroshan Siriwardena. 2011. "Can older people who fall be identified in the ambulance call centre to enable alternative responses or care pathways?" *Emergency Medicine Journal* 28, 3, 3–4.

Spilg, Edward G., Benjamin J. Martin, Sarah L. Mitchell and Tom C. Aitchison. 2003. "Falls risk following discharge from a geriatric day hospital." *Clinical Rehabilitation* 17, 3, 334–340.

The British Pain Society. 2010. Cancer pain management. London: The British Pain Society. www.britishpainsociety.org/static/uploads/resources/files/book_cancer_pain.pdf

Thirugnanasothy, Suba. 2010. "Managing urinary incontinence in older people." *British Medical Journal* 341. doi: 10.1136/bmj.c3835.

Thom, David H., Mary N. Haan and Stephen K. Van Den Eeden. 1997. "Medically recognized urinary incontinence and risks of hospitalization, nursing home admission and mortality." *Age Ageing* 26, 367–374.

Tian, Yang, James Thompson, David Buck and Sonola Lara. 2013. *Exploring the system-wide costs of falls in older people in Torbay*. London: King's Fund.

Touhy, Teris and Kathleen F. Jett (eds.). 2014. *Ebersole and Hess' gerontological nursing and health aging*. Fourth Edition. St Louis: Elsevier.

Victor, Christina. 2011. *Loneliness in old age: The UK perspective. Safeguarding the convoy: a call to action from the Campaign to End Loneliness*. Oxfordshire: Age UK.

Victor, Christina, Sacha Scrambler, Ann Bowling and John Bond. 2005. "The prevalence of and risk factors for loneliness in later life: A survey of older people in Great Britain." *Ageing and Society* 25, 357–375.

Wagg, Adrian, Jonathan Potter, Penny Peel, Penny Irwin, Derek Lowe and Michael Pearson. 2007. "National audit of continence care for older people: Management of urinary incontinence." *Age and Ageing* 37, 1, 39–44.

Wethington, Elaine and Karl Pillemer. 2014. "Social isolation among older adults." In: *Handbook of solitude: Psychological perspectives on social isolation, social withdrawal, and being alone*, edited by Robert J. Coplan and Julie Bowker, 242–260. Malden: Wiley-Blackwell.

Williams, Kate, Phil Assassa, Nicola J. Cooper, Christopher Mayne, Carol Jagger, Ruth Matthews, Michael Clarker and Catherine W. McGrother. 2005. "Clinical and cost-effectiveness of a new nurse-led continence service: A randomised controlled trial." *British Journal of General Practice* 55, 696–703.

Windle, Karen, Jennifer Francis and Caroline Coomber. 2011. "Research Briefing 39: Preventing loneliness and social isolation: Interventions and outcomes." London: SCIE. www.scie.org.uk/ publications/ briefings/briefing39/

Windsor, Julie, Mike Lowry and Sarah Ashelford. 2016. "Orthostatic hypotension 1: Effect of orthostatic hypotension on falls risk." *Nursing Times* 112, 43/44, 11-13. www.nursingtimes.net/clinical-archive/ vital-signs/orthostatic-hypotension-1-effectof-orthostatic-hypotension-on-falls-risk/7013075.article (Accessed 25 April 2017).

World Health Organization. 2008. "WHO global report on falls prevention in older age." Geneva: World Health Organization.

Yu, Michael S., Chetwyn C.H. Chan and Robin K. Tsim. 2007. "Usefulness of the elderly mobility scale for classifying residential placements." *Clinical Rehabilitation* 21, 12, 1114-1120.

7 Frailty and comprehensive geriatric assessment

Samuel Searle and Ken Rockwood

Introduction

Everyone as they get older is closer to death but not every person of the same age has the same risk of death. Variability in the risk of death of people of the same age is frailty (Clegg et al. 2013). Variability in the risk of death. What does this mean? Take ten people who are 80 years old. Let us say they will live on average seven years. This average pertains to the group of 80-year olds but not necessarily to each individual. Some people would be expected to live a year or two, and some others would be expected to live another decade. Variability in the rate of ageing increases with age, and therefore, so does frailty. That is because the longer a group of people lives, then the more time they have to age at varying rates. Individuals who are 50 years old have had 50 years to age differently while 80-year olds have had 80 years. This creates a wider and wider variability in the risk of death of the individual as there is a wide range of ways to age. This variability is reflected in the varying degrees to which people are frail.

In general, people are frail when they have a lot wrong with them, or more technically, when they have accumulated a lot of deficits. For this reason, a comprehensive approach to assessing their health deficits is needed. In addition, the more things that they have wrong with them, the more likely they are not just to be frail, but to also be disabled, and/or have impaired mobility. Mobility and change therein can be a pragmatic way to screen for frailty (Eeles and Low Choy 2015).

A widely viewed YouTube video illustrates the dilemma that faces many older adults when they go to hospital (www.youtube.com/watch?annotation_id=annotation_1685917539&feature=iv&src_vid=IOTVbhHdg4A&v=Fj_9HG_TWEM). Older adults with complex needs are typically not well served by our current systems that focus on providers needs and require patients to present in a "one thing wrong at once' manner. In the video, Mrs A, an independent woman, living with her husband at home presents on a Friday with a fall to the emergency department. She is found to be dehydrated and to potentially have a urinary tract infection. She is admitted and treated with antibiotics. On Monday the health-care team reviews her medical status. Her husband informs the care team she has had progressive problems with her walking and some memory troubles. Physiotherapy assesses her for the next three days, and her medications are simplified. By Wednesday, she is moved to another ward for further rehabilitation as her bed is needed for new acute-care patients. Unfortunately, in the new location she is more confused, falls and sprains her wrist. The following week she is deemed to have no rehabilitation potential and five days later is discharged home with increased support. Unfortunately, she continues to fall and her memory declines further. Her husband suffers from increasing caregiver stress, and she is admitted to a long-term care facility.

Not all countries have, as in the UK system in this clip, an intermediate or subacute-care ward for people to be transferred to once they are discharged from acute-care services. Intermediate care in the United Kingdom most closely, as in this example, approximates to an in-hospital rehabilitation service. Intermediate care-services are sometimes referred to as 'step-down' (e.g. from acute care to rehabilitative) or 'step-up' (e.g. from home to rehabilitative/more acute care).

Even when intermediate-care facilities are available they might not always be used successfully (Elbourne et al. 2013), instead being used, for example, as an acute-medical unit with a level of monitoring somewhere between a hospital ward and an intensive care unit.

Intermediate care is used to reflect many types of different services so check what is really being provided before making any assumptions about the range of services available.

Frailty shapes and directs the care needs of older adults, making it a key concept in contemporary health care, in which many patients are aged 65 years and older. Identification of frailty in an individual is one of the first steps in developing a care plan, and so serves as the backdrop to interdisciplinary collaborative practice. Take a look at Mrs A prior to her first presentation to the hospital. She had a 'herald health' event in her first fall. Had she been identified as frail; her medications might have been adjusted to limit future falls. Physiotherapy services could have been enlisted to help strengthening and balance. Maybe foot care could have been of benefit. A home occupational therapy assessment could have been performed to determine whether there were home modifications in order to improve accessibility and reduce the risk of future falls (see Chapter 6).

Frailty has wide ramifications all across health care (Vermeiren et al. 2016). It impacts health issues, disability, psychological factors, living environments, care networks, and health-care costs. Understanding frailty enables health-care workers to bring context to older adult's health status and what might be involved in day-to-day care or future health trajectories. In this way when someone is labelled as moderately frail, health-care team members have a way to understand and communicate potential needs of the individual in developing a care plan or other health intervention (Turner and Clegg 2014).

Mr G is a 76-year man, dependent on a walking frame for ambulation, who enters a clinic room of his primary-care nurse practitioner. His wife is concerned about his memory. He says he is depressed. He has had a long history with the health-care system. A former smoker who developed chronic obstructive pulmonary disease (COPD) earlier in life and quit after he had a heart attack at the age of 57. He required bypass surgery but was able to return to work with accommodations after a period of short-term disability. He was also diagnosed with atrial fibrillation. He had a transient ischemic attack/'mini stroke' ten years after his heart attack. Six months ago, he had a stroke causing right-sided hemiplegia but due to early recognition and intervention, he was discharged home with only subtle residual right-sided weakness.

A person does not need to be old to be frail and conversely not all old people are frail. Although frailty is seen mostly in older individuals, it extends across the life course (Rockwood et al. 2011, 2017). Modern health and social care have allowed acute illnesses to develop into chronic co-morbidity and disability. In consequence, it may very well be that past successes in single-system diseases and increased longevity have led to a growing population of frail individuals. Mr G is such an example of these successes of single-system health care. His health was well managed with his COPD. Successful management for his heart attack and then stroke allowed him to respond well to the acute illness. The problem here occurs when his chronic conditions and health issues lead him to have a slow or even stepwise decline in his overall function and activity. The prevalence of frailty increases with age across the life course—i.e. it is not just seen in older adults—and by age 85, about half of people are frail.

Defining frailty and recognising it clinically

Frailty, the noun is easy to recognise as unmeasured heterogeneity in risk—here, the risk for adverse health outcomes of people of the same age. Recall, again, that some people who are 80 years old are younger than other 80-year olds. The clinical translation of the adjective (just how do we go about answering "Is this person frail?") is not as straightforward. In general, frailty refers to factors intrinsic to the individual; usually factors related to the social environment, and social determinants of health are referred to separately (e.g. as 'social vulnerability' or even 'social frailty'). All clinical operational definitions of frailty seek to (and typically do) identify individuals who are more prone to adverse outcomes across a variety of inpatient, outpatient, and medical or surgical settings. In this way frailty is generalisable and impacts almost all of adult health care.

Across these many settings, operational definitions of frailty identify individuals at risk for a range of adverse health outcomes. People who are frail are more likely, when acutely unwell, to demonstrate the 'geriatric giants' such as functional decline, falls, cognitive impairment, urinary incontinence, and depression (Clegg et al. 2013). In large population-based studies, frailty predicts osteoporosis, heart disease, dementia, disability, loss of partial or full dependence, health-care use, institutionalisation, and mortality. Frailty also appears to have many organ-specific interactions such as with malignancies, heart disease, and back pain.

Frailty has long been seen as synonymous with loss of physiological reserve. The deficit accumulation approach to frailty aims to unify what is seen clinically to a series of deficits gathered on a subcellular level, progressing to the level of cells, tissues, and eventually organ systems before presenting as something clinically identifiable (Rutenberg et al. 2017). Early work is done identifying these preclinical markers (Howlett et al. 2014). This has ramifications for public health, health promotion, and preventative medicine as there may be a way to target individuals before they become frail. This is helping to inform patient health trajectories in both inpatient and outpatient settings, and specifically help to inform how acute illness outcomes can be predicted by frailty. For instance, Mr K is an 84-year-old living in a long-term care facility, dependent on personal care, wheelchair dependent, and has Parkinson's disease. Recently you had noted he appeared pale, and it was found he had anaemia. He is started on iron and he seems to be symptom free (no fatigue, no abdominal symptoms). Usually he would be investigated for a colon cancer but after a discussion with Mr K and his family, it is decided to take a watchful-waiting approach. The long-term care facility staff are made aware of symptoms and signs to monitor. In Mr K's case, identifying his level of frailty, which appears to be in the severe range, gives a tentative prognosis for life expectancy and cautions what types of intervention would result in meaningful quality and quantity of life. For instance, if this anaemia represented a colon cancer, it is known that for a colon cancer to develop it can take up to 10 years. How likely is this potential cancer to impact his length or quality life? If he had further investigations or interventions what would be the pros and cons impacting his length and quality of life? What are his goals? This approach represents person-centred, respectful care.

It is also important to understand what is sometimes misidentified as frailty. Frailty is not simply co-morbidity or disability, although more often than not, these will be present in people who are frail—and when that happens, the more they are present, the frailer an individual will be (Theou et al. 2012). It is not exclusively associated with any of sarcopenia (muscle wasting and weakness), disability, or cognitive impairment, even though someone who had all of these would be frail. How frailty is related to 'normal' ageing and whether it arises in everyone who lives long enough, which seems likely, is not entirely clear.

Measuring and assessing frailty

Comprehensive geriatric assessment

As the global population ages, it is the professional responsibility of nurses, and the other members of the multidisciplinary team, to familiarise themselves with the various tools used within their workplace to assess frailty. The highest standard for identifying frailty has always been considered a comprehensive geriatric assessment (CGA) (an example CGA form is seen in Figure 7.1). This is a thorough, multisystem evaluation of such factors as cognition, emotional status, self-rated health, communication (information 'in' and 'out'), mobility, falls and their contributing factors, bowel/bladder function, nutrition and weight changes, activities of daily living, sleep, co-morbidities and associated medications, and social support and circumstances. In this current form of the CGA, appropriate boxes would be checked off (i.e. hearing, 'WNL' for within normal limit or 'impaired') or ability circled (i.e. dressing, 'ind' for independent, 'asst' for assist, and 'dep' for dependent). The team effort involved in intricacies and management of these domains is at the heart of geriatric medicine.

A CGA must document an individual's baseline health status (not just at a time point where acute medical issues are active). Typically, this can be done most feasibly by finding out, precisely, about each area two weeks prior to the acute illness. Doing so conforms to the general proposition that it is hard to make people better than they were two weeks before they became ill. In Figure 7.1, the domains balance, mobility, nutrition, elimination, and activities of basic living (IADLs, ADLs) all can be assessed at current level as well as two weeks prior to assessment. Not only does this give an understanding of baseline health but also focuses on how much their health has acutely declined with their current acute illness. Information can come from a variety of sources. When cognitive impairment is present, a collateral history is necessary to get valid information on health issues and function.

Capital Health

Comprehensive Geriatric Assessment Form

WNL = Within Normal Limits   ASST = Assisted
IND = Independent   DEP = Dependant

		BASELINE (two weeks ago)				CURRENT (today)				
○ **Cognitive Status**		□ WNL □ CIND/MCI Chief lifelong occupation: _____		□ Dementia □ Delirium		MMSE _____ FAST _____ Education: (years) _____				
○ **Emotional**		□ WNL □ ↓ Mood □ Depression □ Anxiety □ Fatigue □ Other								
○ **Motivation**		□ High □ Usual □ Low **Health Attitude** □ Excellent □ Good □ Fair □ Poor □ Couldn't say								
○ **Communication**		**Speech** □ WNL □ Impaired **Hearing** □ WNL □ Impaired **Vision** □ WNL □ Impaired								
○ **Strength**		□ WNL □ Weak Upper: PROXIMAL DISTAL Lower: PROXIMAL DISTAL								
○ **Mobility**	Transfers Walking Aid	IND ASST DEP IND SLOW ASST DEP				IND ASST DEP IND SLOW ASST DEP				
○ **Balance**	Balance Falls	WNL Impaired N Y Number____				WNL Impaired N Y Number____				
○ **Elimination**	Bowel Bladder	CONT CONSTIP INCONT CONT CATHETER INCONT				CONSTIP CONT INCONT CATHETER CONT INCONT				
○ **Nutrition**	Weight Appetite	GOOD UNDER OVER OBESE WNL FAIR POOR				STABLE LOSS GAIN WNL FAIR POOR				
○ **ADLs**	Feeding Bathing Dressing Toileting	IND ASST DEP IND ASST DEP IND ASST DEP IND ASST DEP				IND ASST DEP IND ASST DEP IND ASST DEP IND ASST DEP				
○ **IADLs**	Cooking Cleaning Shopping Medications Driving Banking	IND ASST DEP IND ASST DEP IND ASST DEP IND ASST DEP IND ASST DEP IND ASST DEP				IND ASST DEP IND ASST DEP IND ASST DEP IND ASST DEP IND ASST DEP IND ASST DEP				

NOTES (right column of table)

Patient contact (Pt.):
□ Inpatient
□ Clinic
□ GDH
□ NH
□ Outreach
□ Home
□ Assisted living
□ ER
□ Other

How many month since well?

Current Fraity Score:

Scale	Pt.	CG
1. Very fit		
2. Well		
3. Well c̄ Rx'd co-morbid disease		
4. Apparently vulnerable		
5. Mildly frail		
6. Moderately frail		
7. Severely frail		
8. Very severely ill		
9. Terminally ill		

○ **Sleep** □ Normal   □ Disrupted   □ Daytime drowsiness   **Socially Engaged** □ Freq □ Occ □ Not

○ **Social**
□ Married
□ Divorced
□ Widowed
□ Single
□ Advance directive in place?

Lives
□ Alone
□ Spouse
□ Other

Home
□ House (Levels ___)
□ Steps (Number___)
□ Apartment
□ Assisted living
□ Nursing home
□ Other

Supports
□ Informal
□ HCNS
□ Other
□ Req. more support
□ None

Caregiver relationship
□ Spouse
□ Sibling
□ Offspring
□ Other

Caregiver Stress
□ None
□ Low
□ Moderate
□ High

Caregiver occupation: (CG)

○ **Code Status** □ Do not resuscitate □ Resuscitate

Problems: Med adjust req.   Associated Medication: (*mark meds started in hospital with an asterisks)
1. _____ ○ _____
2. _____ ○ _____
3. _____ ○ _____
4. _____ ○ _____
5. _____ ○ _____
6. _____ ○ _____
7. _____ ○ _____
8. _____ ○ _____
9. _____ ○ _____
10. _____ ○ _____
11. _____ ○ _____

ACTION REQUIRED (check appropriate circles)

Assessor/Physician: _____   Date: _____
                                                       YYYY/MM/DD

Assessment Forms

Figure 7.1 An example of a one-page CGA.

In someone with a diagnosis of dementia, the fidelity of the patient's understanding can be uncertain, especially on crucial items such as driving, medication use, and financial management. By contrast, other information such as the presence of urinary incontinence can be more readily verified. Taking a history requires that clinical judgement be exercised; the document needs to reflect the best approximation of the true case. With acute changes (e.g. as in delirium) many aspects of a patient's level of function can change—they will be worse than their normal baseline status. Knowing the baseline status can allow for care planning. This can be as simple as asking the patient or family whether the patient could return home if their function and mobility returned to baseline. Often, acute illness in older adults becomes a tipping point, beyond which recovery is less or unlikely. Knowing whether this is the case requires the baseline state i.e. health status to be known with precision. Especially with frail older adults, sometimes a change in function (or mobility or cognition) is all that points to an acute health issue.

Beyond a CGA, two approaches to measuring frailty can be seen as either a syndromic/phenotypic (Fried et al. 2001) or a health-deficit accumulation approach (Mitnitski et al. 2001). The syndrome approach consists of understanding frailty as three or more of muscle weakness, slowed gait speed, fatigue, weight loss, and low physical activity. One or two items present denotes pre-frail and zero, robust. As described by health-deficit accumulation, frailty is the combined sum, across the life course, of all the health problems. In this approach frailty is better appreciated as a spectrum between robust and frail.

Let us look back at our case of Mr G. This case has so far only emphasised the accumulation of his health problems, mainly through co-morbidities. Taking a closer 'geriatric' view, prior to his heart attack, he was able to work inside and outside of the home and only had one time where he needed to go to the emergency department to have his COPD treated. At this time, he was relatively well but living with co-morbid disease. He was very functional, yet not routinely physically active. During the six months prior to his heart attack and surgery, he was progressively exhausted and held off his usual gardening that year. This period of time shows a progression along the continuum of frailty and would be characterised as vulnerable (having more characteristics of frailty). Following his heart attack and diagnosis of atrial fibrillation, he returned to exercising regularly, though limited by dyspnoea, his energy returned, and he was able to tend to a simple garden. This would appear to represent a better state of health than prior to his heart attack and somewhere between vulnerable and well but living with co-morbid disease. Over the intervening years until his stroke, he managed well, eventually hiring someone for his gardening, outside chores and monthly cleaning inside the house; again progressing but now to mildly frail. His activity level was maintained for a time until he found his osteoarthritis paining him more, and he started to limit his regular walks with his wife. His wife found she needed to repeat herself more. Following Mr G's stroke, he and his wife moved into an apartment and he started using a cane or walker most of the time. Three months following discharge from the hospital, his wife found he was more forgetful, he was uninterested in the finances and no longer wanting to go for walks. In this case Mr G progresses in his overall health status, accumulating health issues, recovering from some when properly managed or treated. Somewhere between his heart attack and stroke, he would be characterised as frail. After he has his stroke, he is even more frail.

The Clinical Frailty Scale

Many community and primary-care tools can screen (and are recommended) for frailty. Such examples are assessments of gait speed (formal or not) (see Timed Up and Go (TUG) test (www.unmc.edu/media/intmed/geriatrics/nebgec/pdf/frailelderlyjuly09/toolkits/timedupandgo_w_norms.pdf), and the PRISMA-7 questionnaire ("Fit for Frailty"- www.bgs.org.uk/campaigns/fff/fff_full.pdf) (see Box 7.1).

Box 7.1 The PRISMA-7 questionnaire

Screened positive for frailty if 'yes' is answered to three or more of the following questions.

1   Are you more than 85 years old?
2   In general do you have any health problems that require you to limit your activities?
3   Do you need someone to help you on a regular basis?
4   In general do you have any health problems that require you to stay at home?
5   In case of need can you count on someone close to you?
6   Do you regularly use a stick, walker, or wheelchair to get about?

Another simple, easily understood tool for summarising the degree of frailty, commonly used in Canada and the United Kingdom is the Clinical Frailty Scale (CFS) (Rockwood et al. 2005) (see Figure 7.2). The CFS aims to grade degrees of fitness/frailty, showing the importance of not seeing frailty as 'all or none'. It assesses mobility, function, and self-rated health. Each of these variables integrates a lot of information, so that people with impairments in any of them typically have accumulated many deficits. The scale takes into account physical activity, disease symptoms, activities of daily living, and dependence. The CFS can be completed from screening information or to summarise the results of a CGA.

Clinical Frailty Scale*

 1   **Very Fit** – People who are robust, active, energetic and motivated. These people commonly exercise regularly. They are among the fittest for their age.

 2   **Well** – People who have **no active disease symptoms** but are less fit than category 1. Often, they exercise or are very **active occasionally**, e.g. seasonally.

 3   **Managing Well** – People whose **medical problems are well controlled**, but are **not regularly active** beyond routine walking.

 4   **Vulnerable** – While **not dependent** on others for daily help, often **symptoms limit activities**. A common complaint is being "slowed up", and/or being tired during the day.

 5   **Mildly Frail** – These people often have **more evident slowing**, and need help in **high order IADLs** (finances, transportation, heavy housework, medications). Typically, mild frailty progressively impairs shopping and walking outside alone, meal preparation and housework.

 6   **Moderately Frail** – People need help with **all outside activities** and with **keeping house**. Inside, they often have problems with stairs and need **help with bathing** and might need minimal assistance (cuing, standby) with dressing.

 7   **Severely Frail** – **Completely dependent for personal care**, from whatever cause (physical or cognitive). Even so, they seem stable and not at high risk of dying (within ~ 6 months).

 8   **Very Severely Frail** – Completely dependent, approaching the end of life. Typically, they could not recover even from a minor illness.

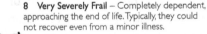 9. **Terminally Ill** - Approaching the end of life. This category applies to people with **a life expectancy <6 months**, who are **not otherwise evidently frail**.

Scoring frailty in people with dementia

The degree of frailty corresponds to the degree of dementia. Common **symptoms in mild dementia** include forgetting the details of a recent event, though still remembering the event itself, repeating the same question/story and social withdrawal.

In **moderate dementia**, recent memory is very impaired, even though they seemingly can remember their past life events well. They can do personal care with prompting.

In **severe dementia**, they cannot do personal care without help.

* 1. Canadian Study on Health & Aging, Revised 2008.
2. K. Rockwood et al. A global clinical measure of fitness and frailty in elderly people. CMAJ 2005;173:489-495.

 DALHOUSIE UNIVERSITY *Inspiring Minds*

Figure 7.2 The Clinical Frailty Scale.

On the CFS, '1' represents the most fit or robust. This would be someone who is very fit for their age group. A typical person would be one who appears to be without health issue and is regularly exercising. A CFS of '2' would also be someone who is well but not regularly active. This could be the older person who is still working outside of the house and staying busy. A CFS of '3' would represent someone who is living independently but could have regular symptoms from a chronic condition such as some dyspnoea with COPD or even paraesthesia from diabetes mellitus. A CFS of '4' would be individuals who are starting to slow down to the point where they are able to be independent but may need to start to use a cane. They may need some help with some of the more physical or even hard to organise tasks routinely done. In mild frailty, a CFS of '5' there may be some problems with daily activities like cleaning the house or cooking meals and/or limited mobility outside of the house. Moderate frailty or a CFS of '6' would generally be exemplified by someone with mobility limited to one floor, unable to do daily tasks outside the home and starting to have some difficulty or limitation with some personal care such as bathing (especially difficult to navigate bath tubs) or dressing (reaching back to put arms in sleeves is often the limitation). Individuals who are completely dependent for personal care like grooming, dressing, bathing, toileting, or even eating are considered severely frail (CFS of '7'). Very severely frail individuals (CFS of '8') are bed bound and unlikely to be able to recover from an acute illness such as pneumonia. On the CFS, terminally ill participants are considered a '9'. A parallel scoring algorithm is offered when this occurs in the setting of cognitive impairment or dementia. Community-dwelling people with moderate to severe frailty (CFS scores '6' or '7') have an approximately 50% mortality rate in just over three years. Of the people who do not die, 40% will be institutionalised and only 25% will still be living in their home (Rockwood et al. 2005). This emphasises the importance of recognising frailty.

Recognising frailty helps in evaluating patients in several health-care settings or presentations. Patients with polypharmacy (on five or more medications), cognitive impairment, a decline in their mobility, or dependent for care, all might be frail. This added recognition might necessitate future management with specialised geriatric care or a more thorough CGA to look at underlying contributing factors. Nevertheless, identifying frailty will allow health-care providers to remain patient centred in approach and assist the care provided. The lack of resilience that goes with frailty means that, against a background of slow decline, disruptions can accelerate the degree of decline, with much less chance of recovery. In a history, this is typically captured by the phrase that someone "has never been the same since" a specific illness or social event. Mr G had been getting gradually frailer over the course of the case presentation. After his stroke, he declined significantly, so much so that his wife could have said "since his stroke, he has never been the same again".

It is important not to misrepresent frailty. Concerning situations for misrepresentation are in the acute or subacute settings. In the critical care setting, everyone looks unwell and everyone who is older, especially with wrinkles or grey hair, looks frail. The intubated 80-year-old woman who at baseline was dependent on personal care, using a walker, with severe stage dementia, looks nearly indistinguishable from the intubated 80-year-old woman who prior to their acute illness was running marathons. Frailty is best assessed at baseline health, as acute illness might distract from the underlying robustness of an individual. The greatest concern in this situation would be the potential for over-representing how frail someone is and rationalising their care. The type of tool used to assess frailty could improperly characterise it. Someone who is unwell could appear looking frail, and if a physical performance tool, for instance, was approximating frailty in this setting, then the physical performance tool could over represent frailty. Such an example could be using gait speed as a proxy for frailty during acute illness. Someone who has decompensated congestive heart failure will have a slower gait speed due to dyspnoea than when medically optimised. If the frailty tool were one such as the CFS, then it would be important to gather information for clinical assessment of the individual when they were last at their baseline. Practically, this baseline is usually two weeks prior to acute illness and can be done by gathering information from a variety of sources.

As people progress through the stages of frailty, their risk for adverse outcomes increases. This becomes especially so when their degree of frailty is such that the factors that allow them to recover become compromised. In other words, as frailty increases, a person's capacity to manage additional health issues becomes even more difficult. An individual who has diabetes mellitus, with an associated chronic kidney disease and foot pain from a diabetic peripheral neuropathy, has a myocardial infarct. The ability to treat and manage this condition may be less as it is not uncommon for neuropathy causing foot pain to limit regular physical activity. Certain medication might need to be dosed according to renal function, not an uncommon adjustment to overlook. At the time of the myocardial infarct, there might also be an acute worsening of renal function. Such scenarios make care of people who are frail more challenging when they become acutely ill. A related challenge is frail individuals are more likely to present not with typical symptoms (e.g. chest pain in myocardial infarction) but with non-specific presentations, such as delirium, or falling or taking to bed. When a fit individual develops an acute illness, they might have a short transient episode of illness resulting in a brief time requiring rest to recuperate. A 30-year-old woman has an urinary tract infection. She has dysuria, suprapubic pain. She goes to work for the day but is less pleasant and social, returning from work as soon as her work is done. She decides to order in for supper and go to bed early. The same illness (or lesser ones such as constipation, dehydration, or even a change in care partner) in a frail individual might result in significant disability beyond their baseline function. Additionally, it takes more time to recover from a given illness and should recovery occur, often times the new baseline health or function is worse than their prior baseline. These ramifications are broad. While individuals might be recovering from illness and slowly improving their function, they will need to be supported and cared for through this prolonged period either in an inpatient or community setting. A moderately frail 80-year-old woman presents to the emergency department with confusion, decreased intake by mouth, and is found, only on examination, to have suprapubic pain and a fever. She is found to have a urinary tract infection and is admitted to hospital. There is a trial of antibiotics and by day two her confusion is resolving while mobility gains are made. Discharge from hospital is five days following admission.

Lessening the risk of hospital-associated deconditioning and disability

A practical approach to managing frail patients starts with recognition of the entity itself and then factors contributing to frailty (Landefeld et al. 1995, Ellis et al. 2017). Managing the individual factors that contribute to frailty contributes to patient- and caregiver-centred care. Such an example could be optimising management of a given co-morbidity tempered with understanding how that might affect mobility, function, or other potential adverse events. Treating to a blood pressure target is important for avoiding health complications such as strokes or myocardial infarcts but if it causes postural hypotension, and falls, not only would this contribute to future risks but can be contributing to worse overall health and function currently. Other important factors, which of course can help anyone at risk, are maintaining adequate dietary requirements, ensuring appropriate support networks, maintenance of mental health, and ongoing physical activity. It appears that even very frail individuals respond to exercise, and exercise may be able to reverse some elements of frailty. Medication reviews cannot be over utilised as many older frail adults have polypharmacy.

In the acute and subacute setting, general principles of managing frail individuals (see Box 7.2) are maintained.

Regular mobility is particularly important. If safe, taking a frail individual for a walk or having them up in a chair are simple mobility exercises that help future function and recovery from acute illnesses. If there is a decline in mobility, this could signify treatment failure or emerging new health problems (MacKnight and Rockwood 2000). Ensuring that bowel movements are regularly occurring is important, as is ensuring adequate nutrition. Older frail adults may have functional limitations, preventing them from eating or doing other functional activities due to the mismatch of their function with the environment. Mrs H is admitted to hospital for pneumonia but has a history of essential tremor. She is fatigued because of her illness. Each time she tries to have a sip of her tea, she spills it over her bed sheets and shirt.

Great attention must be paid to sleep, pain, hygiene, communication with patients and family, and individualised care planning. The fact that hospitals often get away with not doing so in fitter patients is not an endorsement for not doing so in those most in need of such approaches.

Early recognition and management of health issues is important in frail individuals. This is exemplified best by protocols to have early interventions on hip fracture repair.

Box 7.2 General principles of managing frail individuals

- Patient centred goals/Goal attainment
- Rehabilitation/Exercise
- Nutrition/Hydration
- Medication review
- Care planning
- Education.

The sooner a hip fracture is repaired, the lower the mortality and the better the functional outcome. The longer frail individuals are unwell, the more likely they will have a longer recovery with an even lower functional baseline.

A key part of optimal management of frail patients is ensuring care for the carers. Many frail individuals are dependent on others for daily activities. This is true when individuals are recovering from illness, as formerly described, when they are managing with an acute illness, and when they have associated functional impairments on a daily basis. It is important that there is a support network available. This could be formal and/or informal. Beyond this, there are additional social determinants of health important to the frail elderly. Such factors as proper housing, food security, access to health care, income, wider social networks, and ethnicity all impact health and frailty. Social vulnerability enables even further risk of adverse outcomes (Andrew et al. 2008).

One of the great pleasures of caring for older people is understanding that when care is provided to a frail older adult, there is more often than not a network of family and friends who are also benefiting from this care provided. This helps support their own health. Competent and knowledgeable nurses can provide direct care with wide-reaching potential. There are opportunities to educate those being cared for as well as family members on ageing and frailty. In this way, future health decisions can be better made, patients and families can be empowered, and health crises may be recognised sooner or avoided altogether.

Frailty is a clinically important phenomenon, even if perceived as a negative term (Mudge and Hubbard 2017). It is important to consider how this term might impact the patient's perspective. The inverse of this term is robust or resilient, so it would be hard to argue that someone who has lived well into their 90s has not been resilient. It is therefore important to know that often frail individuals have lived a resilient life thus far and their dignity must be paramount.

Summary of key messages

- Frailty is a key concept in older adult care. Being able to recognise and assess frailty while avoiding its pitfalls—missing the phenomenon, over calling frailty in acute illness, failing to make care plans, missing intervening on reversible features, not involving the care network—is important, and is rooted in an approach that embraces the complex needs of frail older adults, through a CGA, and evaluation of high-order functions (mobility, balance, cognition, function, and social interaction).
- Understanding the determinants of frailty helps inform a prevention agenda.
- Understanding the typical health trajectories of frailty (gradual change, often with periods of acceleration around acute illness or social changes) has broad reaching implications for how health and social care need to be organised—including how they should respond.
- Good quality care in frail individuals is specific to the individual.
- In general, focusing particularly on exercise and nutrition and ensuring a strong social support network and education empower patient-centred care and enable older frail adults to avoid adverse health outcomes.

References

Andrew MK, Mitnitski AB, Rockwood K. Social vulnerability, frailty and mortality in elderly people. *PLoS ONE*. 2008 May 21;3(5):e2232. doi: 10.1371/journal.pone.0002232

Clegg A, Young J, Iliffe S, Rikkert MO, Rockwood K. Frailty in elderly people. *Lancet*. 2013 Mar 2;381(9868):752–62. doi: 10.1016/S0140-6736(12)62167-9.Erratum in: *Lancet*. 2013b;382(9901):1328.

Eeles E, Low Choy N. Frailty and Mobility. *Interdiscip Top Gerontol Geriatr*. 2015;41:107–20. doi: 10.1159/000381200.

Elbourne HF, Hominick K, Mallery L, Rockwood K. Characteristics of patients described as sub-acute in an acute care hospital. *Can J Aging*. 2013;32(2):203–8.

Ellis G, Gardner M, Tsiachristas A, Langhorne P, Burke O, Harwood RH, Conroy SP, Kircher T, Somme D, Saltvedt I, Wald H, O'Neill D, Robinson D, Shepperd S. Comprehensive geriatric assessment for older adults admitted to hospital. *Cochrane Database Syst Rev*. 2017 Sep 12;9:CD006211. doi: 10.1002/14651858.CD006211.pub3

Fried LP, Tangen CM, Walston J, Newman AB, Hirsch C, Gottdiener J, Seeman T, Tracy R, Kop WJ, Burke G, McBurnie MA.Cardiovascular Health Study Collaborative Research Group. Frailty in older adults: evidence for a phenotype. *J Gerontol A Biol Sci Med Sci*. 2001 Mar;56(3):M146–56.

Howlett SE, Rockwood MR, Mitnitski A, Rockwood K. Standard laboratory tests to identify older adults at increased risk of death. *BMC Med*. 2014 Oct 7;12:171. doi: 10.1186/s12916-014-0171-9

Landefeld CS, Palmer RM, Kresevic DM, Fortinsky RH, Kowal J. A randomized trial of care in a hospital medical unit especially designed to improve the functional outcomes of acutely ill older patients. *N Engl J Med*. 1995 May 18;332(20):1338–44.

MacKnight C, Rockwood K. Rasch analysis of the hierarchical assessment of balance and mobility (HABAM). *J Clin Epidemiol*. 2000;53(12):1242–7.

Mitnitski AB, Mogilner AJ, Rockwood K. Accumulation of deficits as a proxy measure of aging. *ScientificWorldJournal*. 2001 Aug 8;1:323–36.

Mudge AM, Hubbard RE. Frailty: mind the gap. *Age Ageing*. 2017 Dec 29. doi: 10.1093/ageing/afx193

Rockwood K, Song X, MacKnight C, Bergman H, Hogan DB, McDowell I, Mitnitski A. A global clinical measure of fitness and frailty in elderly people. *CMAJ*. 2005 Aug 30;173(5):489–95.

Rockwood K, Song X, Mitnitski A. Changes in relative fitness and frailtyacross the adult lifespan: evidence from the Canadian National Population HealthSurvey. *CMAJ*. 2011;183(8):E487–94.

Rockwood K, Blodgett JM, Theou O, Sun MH, Feridooni HA, Mitnitski A, Rose RA,Godin J, Gregson E, Howlett SE. A frailty index based on deficit accumulation quantifies mortality risk in humans and in mice. *Sci Rep*. 2017 Feb 21;7:43068.

Rutenberg AD, Mitnitski AB, Farrell SG, Rockwood K. Unifying aging and frailty through complex dynamical networks. *Exp Gerontol*. 2017 Aug 25. pii:S0531-5565(17)30482-5. doi: 10.1016/j.exger.2017.08.027.

Theou O, Rockwood MR, Mitnitski A, Rockwood K. Disability and co-morbidity inrelation to frailty: how much do they overlap? *Arch Gerontol Geriatr*. 2012 Sep–Oct;55(2):e1–8.

Turner G, Clegg A, British Geriatrics Society, Age UK, Royal College of General Practioners. Best practice guidelines for the management of frailty: a British Geriatrics Society, Age UK and Royal College of General Practitioners report. *Age Ageing*. 2014 Nov;43(6):744–7.

Vermeiren S, Vella-Azzopardi R, Beckwée D, Habbig AK, Scafoglieri A, Jansen B, Bautmans I, Gerontopole Brussels Study group. Frailty and the prediction of negative health outcomes: A meta-analysis. *J Am Med Dir Assoc*. 2016 Dec 1;17(12):1163.e1–1163.e17.

8 Living and dying in old age

Catherine Evans and Caroline Nicholson

Our chapter starts with two stories of older people living towards the end of their lives—Mr Wood and Mrs Mathews. We refer to these stories throughout.

Mr Wood is an 88-year-old man with mild memory problems. He comes to the emergency department (ED) with his wife. He has terrible back pain caused by arthritis. He is taking paracetamol, but this gives little pain relief. Mr Wood has attended the ED four times over the last six months because of pain, falling, increasing confusion, and weight loss. His elderly wife, Mrs Wood is finding it increasingly hard to support and care for her husband. Their daughter Sarah lives nearby and is trying to help her parents but works part-time and has a young family.

Mr Wood says: I told the doctor that I never want to go to the hospital again. It's torture—you can't do anything for yourself and you get weaker and sicker. Every time I'm in the hospital it feels as if I'll never get out.

Mrs Wood says: He hates being in the hospital, but what can I do? The pain is terrible, and I can't get the out of hours doctor to call me back. I can't even move him myself, so I call an ambulance. It's the only thing I can do.

Sarah says: I want what Dad wants, which is for him to stay at home. But Mum can't manage when dad is in pain. She doesn't know what to do. It is very distressing for her when she is struggling to get someone to help dad.

Three months have passed. Mr Wood is much frailer. He needs help from his wife to get up from bed, to walk to the bathroom, to wash and dress, and to manage his medicines. He is spending more and more time in bed resting and sleeping. He still enjoys a little food and having his wife close. He is more confused and relies on his wife to explain things and remind him what to do. He attends the ED with his wife because he has a chest infection. His family doctor prescribed an antibiotic, but his chest has little improved. He continues to cough, and his breathlessness is worse. This is the second time in two months that Mr Woods has come to hospital with a chest infection.

Mr Wood says: I told the doctor I didn't want to go back into hospital. It's so tiring and noisy. I don't know who people are and I miss my wife. Each time I go in, I want to get home again, but it gets harder each time to get home. I want to be at home.

Mrs Wood says: I don't know what to do. His breathing is so bad, it is so frightening. I can't get hold of the doctor on the weekend. I don't want him back in the hospital, he hates it, but what can I do? I call the ambulance. It's the only thing I can do.

Sarah says: Mum panics, she always calls the ambulance. Dad saw the doctor and he explained he could stay at home. The doctor explained that Dad might not get better with the antibiotics at home, and that he could arrange for nurses to help look after Dad at home. He also said that Dad could take medicine to help his breathing. That's what he wants, he wants to stay at home with more support, but Mum panics.

(Story adapted from Bone et al. 2016)

Hazel Mathews is a 72-year-old lady with moderate Alzheimer's disease. She has been living in the care home for nine months and moved there when her husband James had a stroke and was no longer able to look after her. James has made a good recovery and visits Hazel regularly. He remains frail however and is no longer able to be his wife's full-time carer. Their children are supportive but live abroad and are only able to visit infrequently.

Functionally, Hazel needs support for most of her personal care needs. She appears to be physically well and has no other illnesses apart from high blood pressure and osteoarthritis. She walks independently and fairly safely although needs some help with transfers at times. Hazel struggles to communicate due to her dementia and at times becomes frustrated when she can't find the right word.

Since moving into the care home, Hazel has generally settled well. She engages in all her personal care needs although requires some encouragement to eat her meals. She is, however, reluctant to take part in any of the activities in the care home and prefers to sit by herself frequently isolating herself in her own bedroom.

Occasionally, Hazel has been observed to be tearful, but no one has been able to ascertain from her why she is distressed. At these times, her communication tends to worsen causing her to become more distressed. Later, when asked, Hazel does not recall crying and seems surprised that she might have been.

Hazel is more cheerful when her husband visits her. When asked why his wife may become tearful, he doesn't know. James has explained that while his wife has always been a little reserved and private, she has been quite easy-going and not easily distressed. He wonders whether she may be in pain and has requested that her general practitioner (GP) visit her.

Three months have passed:

During the past three months, Hazel has been reasonably stable. She continues to have tearful episodes and requires a little coaxing to eat meals and engage. Nonetheless, most of the staff report that they have no concerns regarding providing care. She has had no apparent changes in her health.

James, however, has become quite unwell and had a two-week hospital admission. He is now much frailer and not able to visit frequently. Without close family nearby, he finds it increasingly difficult to get to the care home.

Since then, Hazel has become more withdrawn. She isolates herself frequently and, for the first time, has started to resist some of the care provided. Worryingly, while she has always been a small eater and required some encouragement to eat her meals, she now seems to have lost her appetite entirely. She is losing weight and staff are worried that she may be becoming under-nourished and at risk of dehydration. At times Hazel becomes quite agitated, wandering around the care home. At these times she is very distressed but can't explain why and becomes more distressed and agitated.

(Story adapted from Ellis-Smith et al. 2018)

Introduction

In this chapter we discuss end-of-life care in old age and its integration into living. We emphasise the importance of living as well as possible as end of life nears for the person and their family, and the importance of place of death as well as the nature of death. We draw on the two stories above to illustrate what is important for the person and their families and to apply research evidence to clinical scenarios. We hope that this will help you to understand the challenges of living and dying in advanced age, and the importance of palliative care to enable individuals to live as well as possible and die peacefully.

Older people live increasingly to very advanced ages, and most people in high-income countries die aged 80 years and over. As people live to advanced ages, they commonly live and die with frailty and multimorbidities of two or more long-term conditions (NICE 2016). We will focus on what matters to older people so that they can live as well as possible with frailty and multimorbidities, and their families, and to die peacefully. We will draw on research work to explore the challenges and solutions to enabling older people to live as well as possible in advanced age and emphasise the importance of place of death as well as the nature of death. We draw on the story of Mr Wood and his family to illustrate what matters to the person, how needs and priorities change over time, communication with family, and talking about what is important to enable a peaceful death; Mrs Mathews living with dementia in a care home experiencing increasing symptom distress as her advancing dementia makes it increasingly difficult for her to communicate her concerns. Both stories illustrate the important role played by carers and family members, in providing care and the importance and demands placed upon them.

Living and dying in old age is a mark of societal accomplishment. Increasing longevity presents many joys for an individual, those close to them and society. But living well and dying peacefully can be challenging for all of us. With advancing age many individuals experience increasing health-and social-care needs typically associated with chronic conditions and frailty. However, as needs increase often access to services and the quality of the care provided decreases. There are numerous examples of inequitable access to palliative and end-of-life care and services associated with age from poorer management of cancer pain (Gao et al. 2011), use of aggressive futile treatment in advanced dementia (Mitchell et al. 2009), and lower access to palliative care services compared to younger age groups (Burt and Raine 2006). The causes are many but in order to minimise distress we need to focus on three key points:

1   Societal attitudes towards ageing and older people and the level of priority to attune services to the needs of older people to provide the right care, at the right time, in the right place (Saini et al. 2017).
2   Retaining personhood—being able to tell our story of who we are, communicate 'what matters to me', and for those around us to listen or to advocate and remember for us if we can no-longer because of, for example, cognitive impairment from dementia.

3   The complexity of clinical presentation in old age with increasing number of conditions (multimorbidities) a person lives with, and consequent uncertainty as to the cause of deterioration in health, the presenting symptoms, and the likely outcomes of care of, for example, recovery or continued deterioration leading eventually to end of life (Mishel 1990).

What is essential for nurses is to be compassionate by understanding what matters to the older person and those close to them and aligning care and treatment through shared-decision-making with the older person (and/or those close to them) to pursue individual goals. This requires impeccable assessment that encompasses physical, social, emotional, and spiritual components of health to understand clinical presentation and what matters to the older person as they age and near the end of life.

What is palliative and end-of-life care?

Palliative care is 'everyone's business'; everyone who provides care to people living with life-threatening conditions, including cancer and non-cancer conditions such as dementia, and advanced age, and frailty. Palliative care is patient-centred care in advanced disease, meaning focusing on elements of care, support, and treatment on what matters most to the patient and their family (Health Foundation 2016). The cornerstone is a focus on detailed detection, impeccable assessment, review, and management of multiple domains of health including physical problems such as pain, breathlessness, and mobility; social challenges such as poverty and isolation; psychological difficulties such as depression and anxiety; and spiritual concerns such as existential distress (World Palliative Care Alliance 2014). This needs-based approach allows the person, their carers and staff to focus on living well, maximising comfort, health-related quality of life (QoL), and managing uncertainty, such as nearness to end of life.

What does palliative care mean in old age, and what is the 'added value' of palliative care for people living and dying in old age? This is encapsulated by Cicely Saunders, the founder of the modern hospice movement herself a nurse, social worker, and medical doctor, on the fundamentals of palliative care who stated that:

> You matter because you are you, and you matter to the end of your life. We will do all we can not only to help you die peacefully, but also to live until you die.
>
> (http://www.stchristophers.org.uk/about/damecicelysaunders/tributes)

Palliative care services intend to reduce symptom burden (Gomes et al. 2013) and are value for money in achieving this (Smith et al. 2014). Providing palliative care to older people is recommended in geriatric care and specifically in dementia (van der Steen et al. 2014) but these highly specialised services may not be widely used in practice. Most care for older people is delivered by 'generalist' staff like a GP, community nurse, ambulance, and care home staff. The provision of palliative care forms part of their role and ideally they will have received some training on palliative care. A specialist in palliative care is a practitioner where palliative care forms most of their role and they have received specialist training. Specialists tend to provide care for individuals with more complex needs, for example, overwhelming symptoms (World Palliative Care Alliance 2014). Specialist palliative care teams are multidisciplinary comprising, for example, medical doctors, nurses, physiotherapists, occupational therapists, social workers, counsellors, and chaplains. However, the composition of the team varies by setting, for example, hospital or community, and by country with high-income countries employing specialist consultants in palliative medicine, but in low- and middle-income countries activities may be delivered by, for example, nurses empowered with appropriate training and medical supervision (Knaul et al. 2018).

In old age, a palliative care approach is often started in crisis or when dying is imminent (Sampson et al. 2018), but should be integrated earlier into routine practice by generalist staff, working with specialists for patients with complex needs. The delivery of palliative care is ideally based on individual need and the goal of care to improve quality of life, meaning enabling pursuit of what matters to the person. This is a broader perspective than more traditional approaches of diagnosis such as terminal cancer or prognosis of less than six months.

The emphasis on palliative care in old age for people with advanced conditions such as dementia (van der Steen et al. 2014) is to:

- attend to the **patient's comfort**, meaning health-related QoL by delivering person-centred care that is aligned to 'what matters to me';
- negotiate with a patient about **goals of care 'What matters to me [and my family]'**, and involve in decisions about care and treatment;
- prepare patients for the duality of nearing end of life and undertaking, for example, advance care planning (ACP), while pursuing life-extending/sustaining treatment; and
- manage care and treatment with what seem to be contradictory goals, such as provision of interventions to support recovery and those that anticipate decline such as a 'do not attempt resuscitation' (DNAR) medical order.

End-of-life care is a component of palliative care. The term generally refers to the last 12 months of life with a broader focus than the terminal or dying phase. The term end-of-life care originated from North America and gained use in England, notably through the National End-of-life Care Strategy for Health and Social Care (Department of Health 2008). End-of-life care for older people is defined as:

> End-of-life care for older people requires an active, compassionate approach that treats, comforts and supports older individuals who are living with, or dying from, progressive or chronic life-threatening conditions. Such care is sensitive to personal, cultural and spiritual values, beliefs and practices and encompasses support for families and friends up to and including the period of bereavement.
>
> (Ross et al. 2000, p. 9)

Why are older people 'special'?

Older people are viewed as 'special' when thinking about palliative care for three main factors:

1   Demographic factors—most people die in old age and their numbers are increasing annually across the globe.
2   Illness and condition factors—older people die from very many different causes of death which may be linked to other complex problems such as multimorbidity and social isolation.
3   Environmental factors—older people live and die in many different locations and are often disadvantaged in dying due to inequity in receiving palliative care.

Most people die in old age

Most people who die are aged 75 years and over. In the United Kingdom this group of people account for over two-thirds of deaths, and their numbers are projected to increase particularly in the oldest age groups. By 2040 53% of all deaths in England and Wales are projected to occur in people aged 85 years and over, increasing from 39% of deaths in 2014 (Bone et al. 2017). Overall, deaths worldwide are projected to rise from 57 million in 2015 to 270 million in 2030, with the number of centenarians projected to increase from 317,000 in 2010 to 17.5 million by 2050 (United Nations 2015). These marked changes in our populations have huge implications for health- and social-care services to meet the needs of increasing numbers of people living and dying in advanced age.

Living with multimorbidities and frailty increases with age

What we live with and die from changes as we age. The main causes of death in Europe are diseases of the circulatory system, such as ischaemic heart disease like a heart attack (myocardial infarction), and dementia. In the United Kingdom, dementia is the main cause of death and is increasingly seen as a common co-morbidity, which older people live with alongside of other non-communicable diseases, such as respiratory disease, urinary incontinence, and depression (Poblador-Plou et al. 2014). These types of non-communicable diseases are the main causes of death worldwide (Murray et al. 2012). Patterns of disease change as we live. The group of adults who live to the very advanced ages of 95 years and over typically outlive the chronic conditions, such as heart disease, and cancer, that tend to be terminal for those aged 80–94 years. In very old age causes of death are commonly pneumonia and 'old age', meaning signs and symptoms not defined by a specific disease or condition. Dying forms a picture of increasing frailty and often acute deterioration from a common stressor amongst older people of lung infection, such as pneumonia (Evans et al. 2014). Knowing when end of life is near is often limited to the last days of life. What is important is to understand individual's increased risk to end of life and likely benefit from palliative person-centred care focused on improving QoL.

With advancing age people living with a single disease or condition is uncommon. Layered above a diagnosis of a disease are increasing multimorbidities and frailty (Barnett et al. 2012). Multimorbidity means the presence of two or more long-term conditions (NICE 2016) that can include:

- physical and mental health conditions like diabetes and depression, respectively;
- ongoing conditions such as learning disability;
- symptom complexes such as frailty or chronic pain;
- sensory impairment e.g. sight or hearing loss;
- alcohol and substance misuse.

Older people living with advanced multimorbidity often struggle with multiple changing medications and poor continuity of care between the multiple services they receive which are aligned to single conditions. Discussing palliative care and dying is often neglected with families and the older person, meaning they have limited awareness of the increasing risk of dying. When a crisis occurs, it is often felt as unexpected and ill prepared for (Mason et al. 2016). This quote from an 82-year-old man living with chronic obstructive pulmonary disease (COPD), heart failure, and renal failure illustrates living with multimorbidity:

> Believe you me what between my kidneys and my heart and my lungs they're all working overtime and they're all beginning to show wear and tear which is only right at my age.
>
> (Mason et al. 2016)

An essential aspect of care towards the end of life is optimal management of medicines (called medicines optimisation). This is particularly important for older people with multimorbidity where polypharmacy (taking at least four or five medicines) is common (NICE 2017). Polypharmacy is typically driven by the introduction of multiple medicines for specific health conditions. Medications are prescribed to prevent complications, such as taking statins to lower cholesterol and prevent heart disease; optimally manage a single disease e.g. use of bronchodilators in COPD; and manage symptoms, such as taking analgesia for chronic pain. In England and Wales, it is estimated that 20% of people aged over 70 years are taking five or more medications, and 16% take ten or more medications (Duerden et al. 2013).

In palliative care it is essential to optimise the medications prescribed by reviewing if the risk of harm is greater than the risk of benefit, such as if the burden of taking statins is greater than the likely benefit of preventing cardiac disease for an individual nearing the end of life. Optimising a person's medicines intends to ensure the individual obtains the most benefit from their medicines, and the least harm, such as confusion. What is crucial is to use a person-centred approach to understand what matters to the person and shared-decision-making drawing on the best available evidence to guide decisions, and considering the person's needs, values, and preferences (Greenhalgh et al. 2014). Daily living can often revolve around managing complex medication regimes, particularly in the advanced disease stage. This 'pill-burden' can take time away from pursuing person-centred goals and QoL and increases the risk of drug interactions and harm from treatments (NICE 2017). For example, a range of medicines can precipitate the risk of falling.

Where do older people live and die?

Just as older people live in a variety of settings ranging from their own home to care homes so too do they die across settings, for instance, in their own home, in nursing or residential care homes, in hospitals, or in specialist palliative care settings. Hospital is typically the main place of death for around 50% of the population, but this varies by age, condition, and country. With advancing age, living and dying in a care home becomes increasingly common. In England, around 44% of people aged 85 years and over die in hospital, and 37% die in a care home. Few die at home (16%) (Public Health England 2017). For people with dementia the numbers dying in hospital decrease to around 40%, and those dying in care homes increase to 55%. It is uncommon to die with dementia at home (5%) or in an inpatient hospice facility (0.3%) (Sleeman et al. 2014).

Where older people live and die is dependent on the availability of resources, services, and individual preferences (Abraham and Menec 2016). This leads to variation by region/ state and country. Individuals are more likely to die in a care home due to the greater number of care homes available and the resources to remain there at the end of life (Sleeman et al. 2014). With the right support to meet increasing needs towards the end of life, people for whom a care home is 'their home' typically die there (Public Health England 2017). Living and dying at home is related to community resources, in particular skilled practitioners who know the individual and are available to be called upon during points of deterioration to 'get things done' to enable people to remain in their usual place of care (Bone et al. 2016), and the availability of unpaid carers (e.g. family) (Gomes and Higginson, 2006). Discussing individual preferences with the person and/or family for place of care at the end of life is important to enable individuals to remain in their usual place of care at home or in a care in home (Bone et al. 2016).

As our populations age this will require increase in services at home, care homes and hospitals, and provision of palliative and end-of-life care. In England, by 2040 if current trends continue, the proportion of deaths in the community is estimated to rise to 69% (own residence or a care home), and hospital deaths continue to decrease to 48% (Bone et al. 2017). Reciprocal with this projected increase in deaths per year is the requirement for palliative care, particularly for people with dementia with increasing prevalence associated with advanced age (Etkind et al. 2017).

Continuity of care across care settings is a key aspect within goals of care for older people towards the end of life. Transition between care settings of moving from own residence or care home to hospital is common, particularly in the last months and weeks of life (Sleeman et al. 2018). Mr Wood's story illustrates the reasons why an older person may attend the ED in a hospital, because of acute decline from a chest infection and increasing symptom distress from breathlessness, pain, confusion, and declining mobility. The narrative illustrates how frightening this is for Mr Wood and his wife as his main carer, particularly when she struggles to obtain support from a GP (a family doctor) to visit out of hours (e.g. on a weekend). Figure 8.1 gives an example of transitions in care for an older person with dementia moving between care home and hospital, and the uncertainty surrounding when end of life begins (Amador et al. 2014).

Most people in their last year of life experience at least one unplanned attendance to a hospital ED. The number of attendances often increases in the last months with disease progression and nearness to end of life (Abraham and Menec 2016; Wittenberg et al. 2014). Around 70% of attendance in the last months of life lead to hospital admission, and the likelihood that a person will die in hospital (Smith et al. 2012). For many they would prefer to remain in the familiar surroundings of home or their care home, with sufficient support to feel safe and secure, autonomy preserved and loved ones nearby (Gott et al. 2004). Recognition of palliative care needs such as QoL as the goal of care, and provision of palliative care services such as talking about preferences for care at the end of life and managing symptoms well can reduce people's use of ED in the last months of life (Smith et al. 2012).

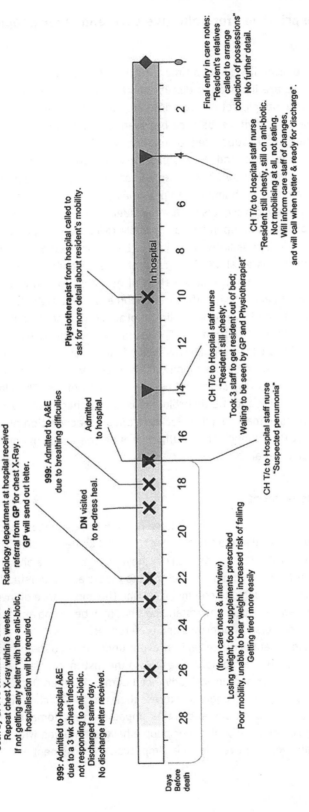

Figure 8.1 Case example of transitions in care last month of life.
Source: From Amador et al. (2014).

What are the priorities for palliative care and older people?

Goal-directed care

Older people have often lived a long time with their conditions. It is imperative that their expertise and goals are included in discussions about future and current care. Evidence suggests that older people retain considerable capability whilst living into late old age (Lloyd et al. 2016). Achieving a balance between loss and continuity is crucial for older people's well-being and is supported, or undermined, by the quality of their interactions with health and social care, and the assumptions that are made about an older person's preferences and capabilities—what they can and cannot do (Nicholson et al. 2012). Goals of care need to encompass both immediate priorities and future preferences and ambitions. Evidence suggests immediate goals of care for older people often centre around remaining mobile and remaining as independent as possible (Nicholson et al. 2018). When an older person could benefit from palliative care is best based on need and intended goals of care of improving QoL (Evans et al. 2019; Mitchell et al. 2004; World Palliative Care Alliance 2014). This moves away from prognostication of nearness to end of life (e.g. 12 months). Judging prognosis is particularly difficult for people with multiple non-cancer conditions, although there are many tools used in clinical practice that seek to indicate requirement for palliative care based on prognosis. For example, the Supportive and Palliative Care Indicators Tool (SPICT) (Boyd and Murray 2010) is available at https://www.spict.org.uk/. When individuals live with multiple conditions uncertainty often surrounds what they may die from and their illness trajectory and nearness to end of life. The illness trajectory for people living with frailty and multimorbidities is often characterised by gradual decline punctuated by points of marked acute decline from an exacerbation of underlying chronic disease, such as COPD (Pinnock et al. 2011), or from a seemingly minor health event like a urine infection (Clegg et al. 2013).

Impeccable assessment

Mrs Mathews' story illustrates her distress and her increasing sadness and withdrawal when symptoms may be under detected and under treated, like her possible pain and loneliness with her husband less able to be near, with her move to a care home and his declining health. The story shows us how challenging it is for staff to assess and understand what is wrong for the person, when they struggle to communicate and the importance of involving people who know them well, like a spouse, in understanding what may be wrong and how best to manage in ways aligned to the person's priorities and preferences.

Impeccable assessment is essential to prevent under detection and under treatment of symptoms, such as pain, that compromise QoL in the last months and years of life. This is particularly important for people with advanced dementia when the severity of cognitive impairment means they will struggle to express their needs (Brecher and West 2016).

Living with multiple conditions and frailty impacts on all domains of health—physical, social, psychological, and spiritual. Older people have often lived with and managed their conditions for many years or even decades. Impeccable assessment and detection of needs and concerns across the domains of health, and person-centred care of understanding and tailoring care to what is important to the person, are cornerstones of both palliative and geriatric care (Evans et al. 2019).

Person-centred care is a core health value of palliative care, geriatric care, and health care in general. Using patient-centred outcome measures (PCOMS) within routine care is a way to enhance the provision of person-centred care by informing assessment, directing care to address priority areas, and measuring outcomes of care, from the perspectives of patients and families, in turn promoting quality and equity (Dawson et al. 2010). Outcome measures used in routine palliative care need to be short because of high fatigue often experienced by patients living with advanced conditions, provide clinically relevant information, be easy to interpret to inform clinical decision-making, be completed by the patient or by someone who knows them well when no longer able to communicate because of, for example, nearness to end of life (Evans et al. 2013). Although use of PCOMS and tools in clinical practice can improve the detection of problems and inform care and treatment, their impact on clinical management depends on how they fit (or not) into routine care (Greenhalgh 2009). The tool needs to be developed with the population they are intended to be used with. This is to ensure they are valid (assess areas clinically relevant and meaningful for the respective condition) and reliable (tool is used in a consistent way by staff).

The Integrated Palliative Care Outcome Scale for dementia (IPOS-dem) is an example of a person-centred measure for palliative geriatric care with clinical validation for use in care homes for people with dementia and multimorbidities (Elis-Smith et al. 2016, 2018). A section of IPOS-dem is detailed in Box 8.1. It comprises ten items and begins with the priorities for the person. The full version for clinical practice is available free at https://pos-pal.org/. The measure intends to enable comprehensive assessment and can be completed by the person or a proxy, for example care home staff. The measure was developed from the established and validated Palliative care Outcome Scale (POS) family of measures (Collins et al. 2015; Schildmann et al. 2015), and is widely used internationally including for low/middle-income countries, for example, the African and Thai POS (Harding et al. 2010; Pukrittayakamee et al. 2018).

Integrated interdisciplinary working across care settings

Older people typically live with many conditions and often over a prolonged period. To maintain well-being and QoL, palliative care needs to support patient capabilities to maintain and optimise function, such as mobility, integrated with problem-solving to manage distressing symptoms and concerns for the patient and their carers. A recent review identified this as a model of integrated palliative geriatric care (Evans et al. 2019). This encompasses palliative care and palliative rehabilitation to engage with both problem-solving that focuses on vulnerability and deficits, such as a symptom like breathlessness, and capabilities to maintain and enhance function, notably a person's mobility.

The overarching goal of care is improving health-related QoL. There is evidence that approaches of both integrated geriatric care with an emphasis on function and integrated palliative care with an emphasis on managing symptoms and concerns can improve QoL

Box 8.1 Integrated Palliative Care Outcome Scale for Dementia v1 extract

POS

IPOS-Dem

Q2. Please select one box that best describes how the person has been affected by each of the following symptoms <u>over the past week</u>.

	Not at all	Slightly	Moderately	Severely	Over-whelmingly	Cannot assess
Pain	0 ☐	1 ☐	2 ☐	3 ☐	4 ☐	☐
Shortness of breath	0 ☐	1 ☐	2 ☐	3 ☐	4 ☐	☐
Weakness or lack of energy	0 ☐	1 ☐	2 ☐	3 ☐	4 ☐	☐
Nausea (feeling like being sick/vomiting)	0 ☐	1 ☐	2 ☐	3 ☐	4 ☐	☐
Vomiting (being sick)	0 ☐	1 ☐	2 ☐	3 ☐	4 ☐	☐
Poor appetite	0 ☐	1 ☐	2 ☐	3 ☐	4 ☐	☐
Constipation	0 ☐	1 ☐	2 ☐	3 ☐	4 ☐	☐
Dental problems or problems with dentures	0 ☐	1 ☐	2 ☐	3 ☐	4 ☐	☐
Sore or dry mouth	0 ☐	1 ☐	2 ☐	3 ☐	4 ☐	☐
Drowsiness (sleepiness)	0 ☐	1 ☐	2 ☐	3 ☐	4 ☐	☐
Poor mobility (trouble walking, cannot leave bed, falling)	0 ☐	1 ☐	2 ☐	3 ☐	4 ☐	☐

but with different emphasis on care delivery (Evans et al. 2019). Taking this forward as a model of integrated palliative geriatric care is a way to align care and treatment, and services to the needs of older people with multimorbidity and frailty. Figure 8.2 overviews key components of a proposed model. This illustrates emphasis on integration between

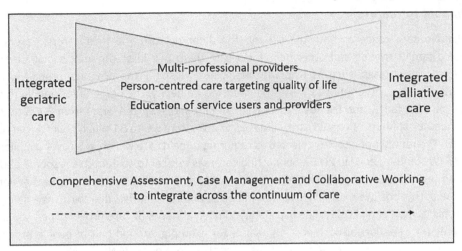

Figure 8.2 Integrated palliative geriatric care and processes to maximise quality of life for older people in the last years of life (Evans et al. 2019).
Source: Adapted from Hawley (2014).

palliative and geriatric care, with the intended goals of care informing service delivery, for example emphasis on palliative care during times of increasing symptoms and concerns, or on rehabilitation with increased geriatric provision. There are examples of these types of approaches such as short-term integrated palliative and supportive care for older people in community settings (Bone et al. 2016), and evidence of rehabilitation intervention giving greatest improvement in muscle strength and mobility for those with the lowest performance associated with advanced COPD (Maddocks et al. 2016). Rehabilitative palliative care intends to optimise capabilities to enable individuals to participate in activities meaningful for them (Tiberini and Richardson 2015). This is an essential approach for older people to support the often long trajectory that they live with chronic life-threatening conditions, and living with dying as conditions progress. What is key to this model is integrating palliative geriatric care in order to manage the continuum of care well. A systematic review on models of care for older people intending to promote QoL identified three proposed key areas (Evans et al. 2019):

1   Comprehensive assessment—meaning a person-centred assessment of needs across physical, psychological, social, and spiritual domains of health. This may use assessment tools for older people like IPOS-dem (Ellis-Smith et al. 2018) or the Comprehensive Geriatric Assessment (see Chapter 7).
2   Case management that focuses mainly on coordination of care for a patient and their carers through the assignment of a case manager: a key practitioner with expertise to assess, coordinate, and review care and treatment.
3   Collaborative working within teams to promote interdisciplinary working, and between organisations such as community services and hospital, to plan and deliver services to meet an individual's health- and social-care needs, as well as their family's needs.

Support for carers

Palliative care concerns both the patient (the older person) and their carers. Carers are unpaid family, friends and other people close to them providing physical, social, practical and emotional tasks, such as help with medicines, washing and dressing, preparing food (Gomez-Batiste and Connor 2017). With increasing longevity, the demand for people to provide care for family and friends is increasing. In England, over ten years from 2005 to 2014 the number of hours of unpaid care increased by 25% from 6.5 to 8.1 billion hours a year (ONS 2016). The number of people projected as requiring unpaid care will grow by over a million by 2035 (Wittenberg and Hu 2015). Supporting carers is critical to sustain this resource and reduce the potentially negative impact of caring on carers' health. Evidence shows that caring can be both a positive experience (O'Reilly et al. 2015) and negative, due to e.g. psychological distress (Simon et al. 2009). The higher the number of hours of care provided per week, the greater the likely negative impact on health. For example, around half of people providing over 50 hours of care per week report their health as 'not good' (ONS 2015).

Assessment of carer support needs is an important part of end-of-life care, particularly to sustain this resource to meet an older person's increasing needs and to enable them to die at home (Gomes and Higginson 2006). The Carer Support Needs Assessment Tool (CSNAT) is a tool developed from evidence and carers and evaluated for community palliative care. The tool and how to use it is available free at http://csnat.org/. The tool includes 14 broad support domains that form two groups: those that enable the carer to care and those that enable more direct support for themselves. The tool is used by the carer to identify the domains in which they require further support. These are then discussed with health professionals. The research work evaluating the tool showed prominent domains as 'knowing what to expect in the future', 'dealing with feelings and worries', and 'having time for yourself in the day'. The tool can be implemented in palliative care practice to improve assessment and management of caregiver needs to ensure adequate support and reduce carer strain (Aoun et al. 2015).

Bereavement

Palliative care is provided to carers until the death of their loved ones and into bereavement. Grief after bereavement is a normal emotional response to loss of a loved one. Grief typically subsides overtime. However, for about 10%–15% of people the symptoms of distress may be more persistent and intense (Latham and Prigerson 2004). Sometimes referred to as "complicated grief" (Shear et al. 2011). Important components for clinical practice are to:

1   Appreciate how care provided towards the end of life and the dying phase impacts on grieving processes, illustrated by a quote from Cicely Saunders: 'How people die remains in the memory of those who live on'.
2   Understand and assess for risk factors associated with complicated grief both before the death to identify carers/family members with increased risk of complicated grief, and post-death at a minimum of six months.
3   Target bereavement resources for individuals with, for example, complicated grief.

Standards for bereavement support in palliative care are available. Work by Hudson et al. (2017) details ten standards and implementation in a bereavement care pathway. The work details risk factors for complicated grief, for example multiple losses sometimes experienced by older people (e.g. the loss of a spouse and siblings in a short period associated with advanced age) and both undertreatment of distressing symptoms (e.g. agitation in the dying phase) and aggressive medical intervention, particularly when futile with little/no benefit (e.g. resuscitation for patients with advanced disease). The stories at the start of the chapter illustrate risk factors of complicated grief in Mrs Wood's increasing experience of caregiver burden and trying to manage her husband's increasing distress, and for Mr Mathews in seeing his wife's increasing withdrawal and growing sadness.

Standards of care detail key principles of assessment to identify individuals at risk of complicated grief, and living with complicated grief, focusing on the primary carer but encompassing other carers/family members, intervention from pre-death and beyond when required, and training and support to palliative care staff undertaking bereavement care (Hudson et al. 2017). Assessment tools are available, with 19 identified as suitable for palliative care, with different tools advocated for different settings and pre- and post-death (Sealey et al. 2015). Although standards and assessment tools are available with evidence of improved outcomes for carers, use in practice is very variable (Hudson et al. 2017). The provision of bereavement support is typically under-resourced and not systematically applied, such as screening patients at six months is rarely established practice in palliative care. This is a vital area for quality improvement to prevent complicated grief and enhance the timely identification and management of complicated grief. To address this gap in clinical practice charitable organisations have grown to provide support and signpost resources, such as Cruse Bereavement Care cruse.org.uk/ and the Good Grief Trust thegoodgrieftrust.org/.

Living and dying in old age

Clinical uncertainty is common and challenging

Whilst there is increasing recognition that many older people will live and die with long-term conditions it is not easy to recognise when to intervene and what care services are most appropriate. Often older people themselves do not always consider themselves to be living with a 'life threatening' long-term condition, and they do not feel it has a significant impact on their lives (Centre for Policy on Ageing 2014). Precisely because people have lived with their illnesses for so long, needs might be overlooked, such as pain or urinary incontinence, because older people (and those around them) normalise these symptoms as part of growing old (Teunissen et al. 2006). It can be hard to recognise life expectancy in older people with multimorbidities and when palliative care might be appropriate. For example, people with dementia can live between 0 and 12 years depending on the type of dementia, stage at diagnosis, and other morbidities that they may live with (World Alzheimer Report 2015). The typical 'frailty' trajectory, first put forward by Lunney et al. (2003), is one of "prolonged dwindling" with the individual living at a low functional level for a period of years, 0–15 years. The lack of a clearly identifiable terminal phase for older people with multimorbidities gives rise to significant periods of uncertainty (Barclay et al. 2014; Gill et al. 2010; Lloyd et al. 2016) and increasing risks to poor outcomes of under assessment and under treatment of symptoms like pain and depression, and aggressive treatment with little or no benefit.

The unpredictable trajectory makes it difficult to diagnose when people are nearing the end of life (Elliott and Nicholson 2017) and increasing vulnerability to sudden health changes means dying may be very rapid. Together these mean that often practitioners avoid discussing with an older person their growing risk of dying, or with their families. The shift from living with to dying from multiple morbidities is often sudden and ill-prepared for so there is little time to prepare or involve the patients and their families in care (Koller and Rockwood 2013).

ACP is important

ACP is important for older people as preferences are typically complex and require skilled professionals to conduct sensitive conversations that are part of an ongoing process (Murtagh et al. 2012). ACP is an ongoing process between a professional and someone nearing the end of life, often with family involvement (Sudore et al. 2017). When imple-mented it decreases inappropriate emergency admissions and invasive procedures, and improves QoL, ensuring care represents the dying person's wishes (Cooper et al. 2014; Jimenez et al. 2018).

However, older people with multimorbidities pose challenges for ACP with often un-certainty as to the nearness to end of life, and/or the likely cause of death, meaning it is often not clear when discussion should begin. Older people's engagement with ACP is often mixed. Preferences for care and place of death are often highly complex, and highly dependent on circumstances that are likely to change over time, notably increasing needs requiring a move to a care home (Murtagh et al. 2012). The illness experience is very differ-ent from that of singular disease such as cancer where often there is clearer understanding of the disease trajectory and nearness to end of life (Kendall et al. 2015).

Symptoms and concerns are common

Both stories illustrate the symptoms and concerns experienced by older people with ad-vanced conditions. Mr Wood's story details living with physical symptoms of pain, breathless-ness, and declining mobility and how these increase overtime and impact on psychological well-being by increasing anxiety for him and his wife. Mrs Mathews' story also details the link-age between the psychological distress of withdrawal and sadness, with physical symptoms of pain and the challenges of assessing symptoms and concerns for people with dementia and a declining ability to communicate their concerns. The last months of life are often asso-ciated with increasing symptoms and concerns associated with advanced disease. The types of symptoms experienced and their severity are similar between cancer and non-cancer conditions (Moens et al. 2014; Solano et al. 2006). The most common symptoms that oc-cur across conditions are pain, fatigue, loss of appetite, breathlessness, and worry (anxiety) (Moens et al. 2014). Key symptoms and concerns specifically in old age are pain, breathless-ness, psychological distress (e.g. anxiety and depression), spiritual distress, incontinence, and fatigue (Age UK 2017). There is a strong association between age and depression, and good evidence on management for people with advanced conditions and effectiveness of treatments such as antidepressants (Rayner et al. 2010).

A key consideration for clinical practice is to ensure adequate assessment and treatment of symptoms and concerns. Under assessment and under treatment of symptoms and concerns can be common particularly when symptoms and concerns are considered an inevitable feature of ageing, overlooking conditions the individual lives with. Poor management compromises individuals' QoL. Assessment can often be hampered because of challenges of limited communication for people with dementia (Mitchell et al. 2009), and a tendency for clinical assessments to focus on a single disease rather than a comprehensive assessment of the person, 'what matters to me' and consideration of the breadth of conditions they live with. Symptom presentation is often complex related to living with multimorbidities, frailty, and disability. These concepts are distinct entities that overlap and impact on each other (Fried et al. 2004). This increases the intricacy of assessing and managing symptoms and concerns to inform management of care and treatment, and the clinical skills and expertise required. National guidance on management of symptoms are important resources to inform clinical decision-making, with best evidence aligned to the priorities and preferences of the individual (Greenhalgh et al. 2014).

Dying well in old age

It is imperative, with the increasing focus of palliative care on life-threatening chronic illness and living as well as possible during this time, not to neglect care of the dying in the last days of life. This is often the time of greatest need (Gomez-Batiste and Connor 2017). National guidance on managing dying are useful resources with recommendations aligned to individual preferences and priorities (NICE 2015). This is particularly important for older people where there are many reports on how care in the dying phase is suboptimal (Parliamentary and Health Service Ombudsman 2015). Older people are less likely to be involved in decisions about their care and treatment, less likely to die where they choose, and are less likely to receive specialist palliative care or access hospice beds (Gott et al. 2011; Seymour et al. 2007; Gott et al 2011).

Poor recognition of nearness to end of life, and likely benefit from palliative care can compromise management of the dying phase with little preparation to enable individuals to die peacefully and in comfort in familiar surroundings. Poor care was characterised by the Parliamentary and Health Service Ombudsman (2015) as having:

- little recognition of dying and continuation of, for example, aggressive treatments with little benefit, such as invasive procedures like taking blood;
- minimal response to needs such as increasing worry and distress;
- poor symptom control; and
- poor communication with families about what is happening.

Summary of key messages

- Palliative care and ageing focuses on the provision of integrated palliative geriatric care. This requires delivery by all those involved in caring for older people across settings in health and social care, notably care homes as the main place of care and death for older people, particularly those with dementia.

- We need to attend to individuals' comfort as well as their capabilities to optimise and maintain function, notably mobility. This is important given the often long length of time older people live with chronic life-threatening conditions to enable them to live life as well as possible and to die eventually in comfort and at peace.
- Palliative care concerns the provision of person-centred care. Emphasis is placed on negotiating with patients about goals of care 'what matters to me', individuals' priorities and preferences, with consideration of the family.
- We need to work with older people to prepare them for the duality of nearing end of life by offering opportunities to engage with ACP, while pursuing life extending or sustaining treatment to ensure optimal management of, for example, chronic conditions. This requires us to manage care and treatment with what often seem contradictory goals at times supporting recovery from an acute event like an infection, while anticipating decline and planning future care.
- Palliative care for older people forms one of the most complex and important areas of clinical practice to enable individuals to pursue their goals and plan for future care towards the end of life to enable individuals to die peacefully and in comfort.

References

Abraham, S., and Menec, V. (2016). Transitions between care settings at the end of life among older home-care recipients: a population-based study. *Gerontol Geriatr Med*, 2. DOI: 10.1177/2333721416684400.

Age UK. (2017). *Briefing: Health and care of older people in England 2017*. London: Age UK.

Amador, S., Goodman, C., King, D., et al. (2014). Exploring resource use and associated costs in end-of-life care for older people with dementia in residential care homes. *Int J Geriatr Psychiatry*, 29(7): 758-66. DOI: 10.1002/gps.4061.

Aoun, S.M., Grande, G., Howting, D., et al. (2015). The impact of the carer support needs assessment tool (CSNAT) in community palliative care using a stepped wedge cluster trial. *PLoS One*, 10(4): e0123012.

Barclay, S., Froggatt, K., Crang, C., et al. (2014). Living in uncertain times: trajectories to death in residential care homes. *Br J Gen Pract*, 64(626): e576-83.

Barnett, K., Mercer, S.W., Norbury, M., et al. (2012). Epidemiology of multimorbidity and implications for health care, research, and medical education: a cross-sectional study. *Lancet*, 380(9836): 37-43.

Bone, A.E., Gao, W., Gomes, B., et al. (2016). Factors associated with transition from community settings to hospital as place of death for adults aged 75 and older: a population-based mortality follow-back survey. *J Am Geriatr Soc*. DOI: 10.1111/jgs.14442.

Bone, A.E., Gomes, B., Etkind, S.N., et al. (2017). What is the impact of population ageing on the future provision of end-of-life care? Population-based projections of place of death. *Palliat Med*. DOI: 10.1177/0269216317734435.

Bone, A.E., Morgan, M., Maddocks, M., et al. (2016). Developing a model of short-term integrated palliative and supportive care for frail older people in community settings: perspectives of older people, carers and other key stakeholders. *Age Ageing*. DOI: 10.1093/ageing/afw124.

Boyd, K., and Murray, S.A. (2010). Recognising and managing key transitions in end of life care. *BMJ*, 341: c4863.

Brecher, D.B., and West, T.L. (2016). Under recognition and undertreatment of pain and behavioral symptoms in end-stage dementia. *Am J Hosp Palliat Care*, 33(3): 276-80.

Burt, J., and Raine, R. (2006). The effect of age on referral to and use of specialist palliative care services in adult cancer patients: a systematic review. *Age Ageing*, 35(5): 469-76.

Centre for Policy on Ageing. (2014). The care and support of older people – an international perspective; a rapid review. www.cpa.org.uk/information/reviews/CPA-Rapid-Review-The-care-and-support-of-older-people-an-international-perspective.pdf (accessed May 2019).

Clegg, A., Young, J., Iliffe, S., et al. (2013). Frailty in elderly people. *Lancet*, 381(9868): 752-62.

Collins, E.S., Witt, J., Bausewein, C., et al. (2015). A Systematic review of the use of the palliative care outcome scale and the support team assessment schedule in palliative care. *J Pain Symptom Manage*, 50(6): 842–53: e19.

Cooper, C., O'Cathain, A., Hind, D., et al. (2014). Conducting qualitative research within Clinical Trials Units: avoiding potential pitfalls. *Contemp Clin Trials*, 38(2): 338–43.

Dawson, J., Doll, H., Fitzpatrick, R., et al. (2010). The routine use of patient reported outcome measures in healthcare settings. *BMJ*, 340: c186.

Department of Health. (2008). *End of life care strategy – promoting high quality care for adults at the end of life*. London: Crown.

Duerden, M., Avery, T., and Payne, R. (2013). *Polypharmacy and medicines optimisation. Making it safe and sound*. London: The King's Fund.

Elliott, M. and Nicholson, C. (2017). A qualitative study exploring use of the surprise question in the care of older people: perceptions of general practitioners and challenges for practice. *BMJ Support Palliat Care*, 7(1): 32–8.

Ellis-Smith, C., Evans, C.J., Murtagh, F.E., et al. (2016). Development of a caregiver-reported measure to support systematic assessment of people with dementia in long-term care: the Integrated palliative care outcome scale for dementia. *Palliat Med*. DOI: 10.1177/0269216316675096.

Ellis-Smith, C., Higginson, I.J., Daveson, B.A., et al. (2018). How can a measure improve assessment and management of symptoms and concerns for people with dementia in care homes? A mixed-methods feasibility and process evaluation of IPOS-Dem. *PLoS One*, 13(7): e0200240.

Etkind, S.N., Bone, A.E., Gomes, B., et al. (2017). How many people will need palliative care in 2040? Past trends, future projections and implications for services. *BMC Med*, 15(1): 102.

Evans, C.J., Benalia, H., Preston, N.J., et al. (2013). The selection and use of outcome measures in palliative and end-of-life care research: the MORECare International Consensus Workshop. *J Pain Symptom Manage*. DOI: 10.1016/j.jpainsymman.2013.01.010.

Evans, C.J., Ho, Y., Daveson, B.A., et al. (2014). Place and cause of death in centenarians: a population-based observational study in England, 2001 to 2010. *PLoS Med*, 11(6): e1001653.

Evans, C.J., Ison, L., Ellis-Smith, C., et al. (2019). Service delivery models to maximize quality of life for older people at the end of life: a rapid review. *Milbank Quarterly*, 97(1): 113–75.

Fried, L.P., Ferrucci, L., Darer, J., et al. (2004). Untangling the concepts of disability, frailty, and comorbidity: implications for improved targeting and care. *J Gerontol A Biol Sci Med Sci*, 59(3): 255–63.

Gao, W., Gulliford, M., and Higginson, I.J. (2011). Prescription patterns of analgesics in the last 3 months of life: a retrospective analysis of 10202 lung cancer patients. *Br J Cancer*, 104(11): 1704–10.

Gill, T.M., Gahbauer, E.A., Han, L., et al. (2010). Trajectories of disability in the last year of life. *N Engl J Med*, 362(13): 1173–80.

Gomes, B., Calanzani, N., Curiale, V., et al. (2013). Effectiveness and cost-effectiveness of home palliative care services for adults with advanced illness and their caregivers. *Cochrane Database Syst Rev*, (6): CD007760.

Gomes, B., and Higginson, I.J. (2006). Factors influencing death at home in terminally ill patients with cancer: systematic review. *BMJ*, 332(7540): 515–21.

Gomez-Batiste, X., and Connor, S. (2017). *Building integrated palliative care programs and services*. Catalonia: Worldwide Hospice Palliative Care Alliance.

Gott, M., Ingleton, C., Bennett, M.I., et al. (2011). Transitions to palliative care in acute hospitals in England: qualitative study. *BMJ*, 342: d1773.

Gott, M., Seymour, J., Bellamy, G., et al. (2004). Older people's views about home as a place of care at the end of life. *Palliat Med*, 18(5): 460–7.

Greenhalgh, J. (2009). The applications of PROs in clinical practice: what are they, do they work, and why? *Qual Life Res*, 18(1): 115–23.

Greenhalgh, T., Howick, J., and Maskrey, N. (2014). Evidence Based Medicine Renaissance G. Evidence based medicine: a movement in crisis? *BMJ*, 348: g3725.

Harding, R., Selman, L., Agupio, G., et al. (2010). Validation of a core outcome measure for palliative care in Africa: the APCA African Palliative Outcome Scale. *Health Qual Life Outcomes*, 8: 10.

Hawley, P.H. (2014). The bow tie model of 21st century palliative care. *Journal of Pain and Symptom Management*, 47(1): e2–e5.

Health Foundation. (2016). *Person-centred care made simple; What everyone should know about person-centred care*. London: the Health Foundation.

Hudson, P., Hall, C., Boughey, A., et al. (2018). Bereavement support standards and bereavement care pathway for quality palliative care. *Palliat Support Care,* 16(4): 375-87.

Jimenez, G., Tan, W.S., Virk, A.K., et al. (2018). Overview of systematic reviews of advance care planning: summary of evidence and global lessons. *J Pain Symptom Manage,* 56(3): 436-59 e25.

Knaul, F.M., Farmer, P.E., Krakauer, E.L., et al. (2018). Alleviating the access abyss in palliative care and pain relief-an imperative of universal health coverage: the Lancet Commission report. *Lancet,* 391(10128): 1391-454.

Kendall, M., Carduff, E., Lloyd, A., et al. (2015). Different experiences and goals in different advanced diseases: comparing serial interviews with patients with cancer, organ failure, or frailty and their family and professional carers. *J Pain Symptom Manage,* 50(2): 216-24.

Koller, K., and Rockwood, K. (2013). Frailty in older adults: implications for end-of-life care. *Clev Clin J Med,* 80(3): 168-74.

Latham, A.E., and Prigerson, H.G. (2004). Suicidality and bereavement: complicated grief as psychiatric disorder presenting greatest risk for suicidality. *Suicide Life Threat Behav,* 34(4): 350-62.

Lloyd, A., Kendall, M., Starr, J.M., et al. (2016). Physical, social, psychological and existential trajectories of loss and adaptation towards the end of life for older people living with frailty: a serial interview study. *BMC Geriatr,* 16(1): 176.

Lunney, J.R., Lynn, J., Foley, D.J., et al. (2003). Patterns of functional decline at the end of life. *JAMA,* 289(18): 2387-92.

Maddocks, M., Nolan, C.M., Man, W.D., et al. (2016). Neuromuscular electrical stimulation to improve exercise capacity in patients with severe COPD: a randomised double-blind, placebo-controlled trial. *Lancet Resp Med,* 4(1): 27-36.

Mason, B., Nanton, V., Epiphaniou, E., et al. (2016). 'My body's falling apart.' Understanding the experiences of patients with advanced multimorbidity to improve care: serial interviews with patients and carers. *BMJ Support Palliat Care,* 6(1): 60-5.

Mishel, M.H. (1990). Reconceptualization of the uncertainty in illness theory. *Image J Nurs Sch,* 22(4): 256-62.

Mitchell, S.L., Kiely, D.K., and Hamel, M.B. (2004). Dying with advanced dementia in the nursing home. *Arch Intern Med,* 164(3): 321-6.

Mitchell, S.L., Teno, J.M., Kiely, D.K., et al. (2009). The clinical course of advanced dementia. *N Engl J Med,* 361(16): 1529-38.

Moens, K., Higginson, I.J., Harding, R., et al. (2014). Are there differences in the prevalence of palliative care-related problems in people living with advanced cancer and eight non-cancer conditions? A systematic review. *J Pain Symptom Manage,* 48(4): 660-77.

Murray, C.J., Vos, T., Lozano, R., et al. (2012). Disability-adjusted life years (DALYs) for 291 diseases and injuries in 21 regions, 1990-2010: a systematic analysis for the Global Burden of Disease Study 2010. *Lancet,* 380(9859): 2197-223.

Murtagh, F.E.M., Bausewein, C., Petkova, H., et al. (2012). Understanding place of death for patients with non malignant conditions: a systematic literature review. Final report. Southampton: National Insitute for Health Research Service Delivery and Organisation Programme.

National Institute for Clinical Excellence (NICE). (2004). *Guidance on cancer services improving supportive and palliative care for adults with cancer.* Oxford: NICE.

National Institute for Health and Clinical Excellence (NICE). (2015). *Care of dying adults in the last days of life.* London: NICE.

National Institute for Health and Clinical Excellence (NICE). (2016). *Multimorbidity: clinical assessment and management.* London: National Institute for Health and Care Excellence.

National Institute for Health and Clinical Excellence (NICE). (2017). *Multimorbidity and polypharmacy.* London: National Institute for Health and Care Excellence.

Nicholson, C., Davies, J.M., George, R., et al. (2018). What are the main palliative care symptoms and concerns of older people with multimorbidity?–a comparative cross-sectional study using routinely collected Phase of Illness, Australia-modified Karnofsky Performance Status and Integrated Palliative Care Outcome Scale data. *Ann Palliat Med,* 7 Supplement 3: 164-75.

Nicholson, C., Meyer, J., Flatley, M., et al. (2012). Living on the margin: understanding the experience of living and dying with frailty in old age. *Soc Sci Med,* 75(8): 1426-32.

ONS. (2015). Full story: the gender gap in unpaid care provisions: is there an impact on health and economic position?

ONS. (2016). Household satellite accounts: 2005 to 2014 – Chapter 3: Home produced 'adultcare' services.

O'Reilly, D., Rosato, M., and Maguire, A. (2015). Caregiving reduces mortality risk for most caregivers: a census-based record linkage study. *Int J Epidemiol*, 44(6): 1959–69.

Parliamentary and Health Service Ombudsman. (2015). Dying without Dignity Investigations by the Parliamentary and Health Service Ombudsman into Complaints About End of Life Care. London: Parliamentary and Health Service Ombudsman.

Pinnock, H., Kendall, M., Murray, S.A., et al. (2011). Living and dying with severe chronic obstructive pulmonary disease: multi-perspective longitudinal qualitative study. *BMJ*, 342: d142.

Poblador-Plou, B., Calderon-Larranaga, A., Marta-Moreno, J., et al. (2014). Comorbidity of dementia: a cross-sectional study of primary care older patients. *BMC Psychiatry*, 14: 84. DOI: 10.1186/1471-244X-14-84.

Public Health England (PHE). (2017). End of life care profiles. https://fingertips.phe.org.uk/profile/end-of-life (accessed 10.08.2018).

Public Health England (PHE). (2017). *The role of care homes in end of life care. Briefing 2 – place and cause of death for permanent and temporary residents of care homes*. London: Public Health England.

Pukrittayakamee, P., Sapinum, L., Suwan, P., et al. (2018). Validity, reliability and responsiveness of the Thai Palliative Care Outcome Scale staff and patient versions among cancer patients. *J Pain Symptom Manage*, 56(3): 414–20.

Rayner, L., Price, A., Evans, A., et al. (2010). Antidepressants for depression in physically ill people. *Cochrane Database Syst Rev*, (3): Cd007503.

Ross, M., Fisher, R., and Maclean, M.A. (2000). *Guide to end-of-life care for seniors*. Ottawa: Health Canad.

Saini, V., Garcia-Armesto, S., Klemperer, D., et al. (2017). Drivers of poor medical care. *Lancet*, 390(10090): 178–90.

Sampson, E.L., Candy, B., Davis, S., et al. (2018). Living and dying with advanced dementia: a prospective cohort study of symptoms, service use and care at the end of life. *Palliat Med*, 32(3): 668–81.

Schildmann, E.K., Groeneveld, E.I., Denzel, J., et al. (2015). Discovering the hidden benefits of cognitive interviewing in two languages: the first phase of a validation study of the Integrated Palliative care Outcome Scale. *Palliat Med*, 30: 599–610.

Sealey, M., Breen, L.J., O'Connor, M., et al. (2015). A scoping review of bereavement risk assessment measures: Implications for palliative care. *Palliat Med*, 29(7): 577–89.

Seymour, J., Payne, S., Chapman, A., et al. (2007). Hospice or home? Expectations of end-of-life care among white and Chinese older people in the UK. *Sociol Health Illn*, 29(6): 872–90.

Shear, M.K., Simon, N., Wall, M., et al. (2011). Complicated grief and related bereavement issues for DSM-5. *Depress Anxiety*, 28(2): 103–17.

Simon, C., Kumar, S., and Kendrick, T. (2009). Cohort study of informal carers of first-time stroke survivors: profile of health and social changes in the first year of caregiving. *Soc Sci Med*, 69(3): 404–10.

Sleeman, K.E., Ho, Y.K., Verne, J., et al. (2014). Reversal of English trend towards hospital death in dementia: a population-based study of place of death and associated individual and regional factors, 2001–2010. *BMC Neurol*, 14: 59.

Sleeman K. E., Perera, G., Stewart, R., et al. (2018). Predictors of emergency department attendance by people with dementia in their last year of life: retrospective cohort study using linked clinical and administrative data. *Alzheimers Dement*, 14(1): 20–7.

Smith, S., Brick, A., O'Hara, S., et al. (2014). Evidence on the cost and cost-effectiveness of palliative care: a literature review. *Palliative Medicine*, 28(2): 130–50.

Smith, A.K., McCarthy, E., Weber, E., et al. (2012). Half of older Americans seen in emergency department in last month of life; most admitted to hospital, and many die there. *Health Aff (Millwood)*, 31(6): 1277–85.

Solano, J.P., Gomes, B., and Higginson, I.J. (2006). A comparison of symptom prevalence in far advanced cancer, AIDS, heart disease, chronic obstructive pulmonary disease and renal disease. *J Pain Symptom Manage*, 31(1): 58–69.

Sudore, R.L., Lum, H.D., You, J.J. et al. (2017). Defining advance care planning for adults: a consensus definition from a multidisciplinary Delphi panel. *J Pain Symptom Manage*, 53: 821–832.e1

Teunissen, D., van den Bosch, W., van Weel, C., et al. (2006). Urinary incontinence in the elderly: attitudes and experiences of general practitioners. A focus group study. *Scand J Prim Health Care*, 24: 56–61.

Tiberini, R., and Richardson, H. (2015). *Rehabilitative palliative care; enabling people to live fully until they die, a challenge for the 21st century*. London: Hospice UK.

United Nations. (2015). *World population ageing*. New York: United Nations.

van der Steen, J.T., Radbruch, L., Hertogh, C.M., et al. (2014). White paper defining optimal palliative care in older people with dementia: a Delphi study and recommendations from the European Association for Palliative Care. *Palliat Med*, 28(3): 197-209.

Wittenberg, R., and Hu, B. (2015). *Projections of demand for and costs of social care for older people and younger adults in England, 2015 to 2035*. London: Personal Social Services Research Unit.

Wittenberg, R.L., McCormick, B., and Hurst, J. (2014). *Understanding emergency hospital admissions of older people*. Oxford: Centre for Health Service Economics & Organisation.

World Alzheimer Report. (2015). *The global impact of dementia, an analysis of prevalence, incidence, cost and trends*. London: Alzheimer's Disease International.

World Palliative Care Alliance, Organisation WH. (2014). *Global atlas of palliative care at the end of life*. London: World Palliative Care Alliance.

9 Conclusions

Andrée le May and Heather Fillmore Elbourne

This book is about the health and well-being of older people and how nurses might positively impact on that. It is not a comprehensive geriatric textbook rather we have focused on the key consequences of growing older to exemplify the critical role of nurses at that time of life–be it providing care at the bedside or advice in the consulting room. Regardless of setting or clinical context nurses must ensure that:

- they speak up for older people–either as a group or as an individual;
- older people receive dignified care; to do this, care must centre around the person;
- families and friends are included in care and care decisions to minimise isolation either of the older person or their family member/friend;
- older people are cared for by multidisciplinary teams, and nurses need to form an integral part of these teams;
- companionship and feeling valued is an important aspect of care.

We brought together a range of experts to help you understand better how nurses and nursing care can impact positively on older people and their families. At the end of each chapter is a summary of their key messages. Whilst we hope you will all read these chapters we realise that this is not always possible, so we have brought these key messages together to close this book.

Summary of key messages on the ageing population

- Changing demographics means that there are more older people than ever before in almost every country in the world–older people are the fastest growing demographic cohort in the world.
- Older people are not only living longer but they are living longer with more complex health- and social-care needs.
- There is both subtle and blatant ageism around us all in our work and everyday lives, and nurses need to understand how that might impact on older people and their care, and how to minimise or, preferably, erase ageism by challenging negative stereotypes.
- Increased numbers of older people, with more complex health- and social-care needs, require increased levels of skilled nursing care; however, finding such nurses in sufficient quantities is becoming increasingly challenging.

- Changes to our health- and social-care systems are needed in order to keep pace with the increasing numbers of older adults needing care.
- Nurses, wherever they work, must be able to provide evidence-based, person-centred care and evaluate its usefulness.
- Nurses need to grasp the opportunity to make positive change that will benefit older people and their families.

Summary of key messages on risk taking and risk aversion

- We need to look beyond the risk of physical harm when assessing risks; risks to social and emotional well-being, especially where autonomy is reduced, are often at least as important for older people.
- We need to collaborate with older people and their families if we are to effectively assess, weigh up, and manage risks.
- We can enable older people to 'take (back) control' by giving them information, confidence, and support to problem-solve. They will then work to balance the risks themselves, in order to do the things that matter to them.
- We need to take time to try and understand the purpose of behaviour which seems puzzling; if we can do this, we can prevent many 'high risk' behaviours.
- We have a key role to play in challenging assumptions that older people 'need to be protected', and risk management practices which have become the norm, often for the sake of organisational efficiency.
- We—and everyone else involved—will have an emotional response to dilemmas of risks and rights. We need to be aware of our own responses, and how they might shape our judgement and encourage others to express their hopes and fears too.

Summary of key messages on staying healthy in older age

- Increasing exercise, maintaining mental agility, and continuing social interaction all have the potential to improve older people's health and well-being.
- Each of these activities can be undertaken individually or collectively.
- There are many influences on undertaking activities in older age, and nurses can play an important part in recognising these and helping, in conjunction with other members of the multidisciplinary team, to reduce barriers.
- Nurses, in all settings and roles, can advise older people and their families about ways to improve their health and well-being. To do this, nurses may use motivational interviewing or social prescribing.
- Many older people use assistive technologies to help them live more independently and to monitor their health more effectively—thus helping them to stay healthier. Nurses need to encourage the proper use of these technologies and be able to guide older people in their use or to experts who can help them.

Summary of key messages on common difficulties experienced by older people

- Understanding the common difficulties encountered by older people will assist nurses and other health- and social-care professionals to be attuned to their complexity.
- Many difficulties that older people experience are interlinked and can be challenging to address. Careful assessment, underpinned by sensitive communication and accurate measurement, is critical to their management.
- Nurses need to be active and equal members of multidisciplinary teams in order to ensure that older people receive the best possible care based on every relevant source of knowledge and skill at their disposal.

Summary of key messages on frailty and comprehensive geriatric assessment

- Frailty is a key concept in older adult care. Being able to recognise and assess frailty while avoiding its pitfalls–missing the phenomenon, over calling frailty in acute illness, failing to make care plans, missing intervening on reversible features, not involving the care network–is important, and is rooted in an approach that embraces the complex needs of frail older adults, through a comprehensive geriatric assessment and evaluation of high-order functions (mobility, balance, cognition, function, social interaction).
- Understanding the determinants of frailty helps inform a prevention agenda.
- Understanding the typical health trajectories of frailty (gradual change, often with periods of acceleration around acute illness or social changes) has broad reaching implications for how health and social care need to be organised–including how they should respond.
- Good quality care in frail individuals is specific to the individual.
- In general, focusing particularly on exercise and nutrition and ensuring a strong social support network and education empower patient-centred care and enable older frail adults to avoid adverse health outcomes.

Summary of key messages on living and dying in old age

- Palliative care and ageing focuses on the provision of integrated palliative geriatric care. This requires delivery by all those involved in caring for older people across settings in health and social care, notably care homes as the main place of care and death for older people, particularly those with dementia.
- We need to attend to individuals' comfort as well as their capabilities to optimise and maintain function, notably mobility. This is important given the often long length of time older people live with chronic life-threatening conditions to enable them to live life as well as possible and to die eventually in comfort and at peace.

- Palliative care concerns the provision of person-centred care. Emphasis is placed on negotiating with patients about goals of care 'what matters to me', individuals' priorities and preferences, with consideration of the family.
- We need to work with older people to prepare them for the duality of nearing end of life by offering opportunities to engage with advance care planning, while pursuing life extending or sustaining treatment to ensure optimal management of, for example, chronic conditions. This requires us to manage care and treatment with what often seem contradictory goals at times supporting recovery from an acute event like an infection, while anticipating decline and planning future care.
- Palliative care for older people forms one of the most complex and important areas of clinical practice to enable individuals to pursue their goals and plan for future care towards the end of life to enable individuals to die peacefully and in comfort.

Appendix 1
Stories of the health challenges associated with older age from the healthtalk-on-line website

Rosemary

Rosemary has type I diabetes, asthma, chronic obstructive pulmonary disease (COPD), rheumatoid and osteoarthritis, and hearing impairment; in the past she has had a heart attack, several strokes, tuberculosis, and a collapsed lung. She was 67 when this interview took place. Rosemary is divorced with five adult children. She is a retired domestic worker. Her ethnic background is White British.

Rosemary links her numerous health problems to childhood poverty. She began taking insulin for type I diabetes in her 30s. She went on to develop rheumatoid and osteoarthritis, which cause her main problems—pain and disability. She had a stroke in the 1990s and began taking aspirin. She has had other minor strokes since but never serious enough to be hospitalised. She had a heart attack in 2000. Rosemary also has asthma and COPD and previously had a collapsed lung. She takes eight tablets daily and another weekly.

Rosemary says that overall she would "like to have known more information about everything". When asked, Rosemary states that she prioritises diabetes: "[it is] the main thing and if I could have a miracle and get rid of it, it would be that. The others, you know, you can learn to live with". Managing diabetes takes a lot of time.

Rosemary says that she has a good general practitioner (GP) but he is popular and so "all the patients want to go to him". "He is good and is very thorough". Generally, she thinks that GPs are overworked. She sometimes feels in a quandary with medical advice e.g. when told a new medicine might make her blood sugars high. Her advice for patients is: "[if] there's something specific you want to bring up, bring it up because otherwise it will be forgotten in listening to what the consultant is saying".

Rosemary describes a difficult balance between controlling diabetes and not putting on weight (through eating too many carbohydrates). She has diabetic neuropathy and a blocked artery in one of her legs makes walking difficult. She has been told by doctors that they wouldn't do an operation to unblock arteries, but she recalls no explanation as to why. Rosemary got a mobility scooter as walking everywhere—as she has done all her life—was becoming too time-consuming.

Rosemary feels that she has no "connection" with consultants as she sees a different one every time: "there's no follow on if you know what I mean." She advises patients to help each other with relevant advice and information.

www.healthtalk.org/peoples-experiences/long-term-conditions/multimorbidities/rosemary#ixzz5Xzi2KMbN

Barry

At age 51 Barry had a stroke that affected his speech, hearing, reading, and writing but he remained mobile. Eight years later he was diagnosed with chronic obstructive pulmonary disease (COPD). He also has a condition of the adrenal glands. He is now 67 years old and is married with one adult child. He is a retired bricklayer and education welfare officer. His ethnic background is White.

Barry feels he would have been unable to deal with the aftermath of a stroke without his wife's support. She came into hospital to provide personal care. He criticises hospital nursing and care staff who "lacked the basics" and "didn't have any common sense". Barry suffered from memory loss after the stroke. There followed a period of depression and excessive alcohol consumption. He gets angry and aggressive and feels he has undergone a "total personality change"; he thinks he's now "very right wing" compared to before his stroke. Barry had smoked since childhood but gave up after the stroke.

Barry's COPD is monitored by telehealth whereby his breathing is assessed over the telephone every morning. He uses a portable oxygen cylinder to help him breathe when away from home. He needs a knee operation, but surgeons won't do it because of his medical history, as he would be "too much of a risk". Barry thinks his general practitioner (GP) is "good," although he seems to have no understanding of what it's like to have had a stroke. Barry's medicines haven't been reviewed in the last eight years: "I think they diagnose you and that's the end of the story". He wants to stop taking statins. His wife manages his medicines for him.

Barry attends a Breathe Easy group with his wife. He values the pamphlets and information provided. On dealing with daily life, he notes:

"I want to do things all the time and suddenly I realise I can't. The toilet bowl went wrong yesterday and I bent down, I knelt down to turn off the stop-cock before I phoned the plumber. I couldn't get back up, you know. You think you're alright, you do it and suddenly realise, 'I shouldn't have done that'".

www.healthtalk.org/peoples-experiences/long-term-conditions/multimorbidities/barry#ixzz5XzrOeW4G

Eric

Eric found out he had heart trouble whilst holidaying abroad a few years after he had been diagnosed with diabetes. However, an enlarged prostate causes him most problems, and he has to plan routes with accessible toilets. He has recently discovered he has a stone in his bladder.

Eric is a retired television engineer and sales manager. He is married with two adult children and is 84 years old. His ethnic background is British.

Eric was diagnosed with type II diabetes and heart failure in his late 60s and early 70s. The latter was treated with stents. However, he experiences more everyday problems from an enlarged prostate, which is not cancerous. Two weeks before the interview he was also found to have a stone in his bladder. He experiences constipation, which he attributes to the medicines he is prescribed.

Eric went to a seminar run by a diabetic nurse at his general practitioner (GP) surgery. His wife went with him as she is mainly responsible for his diet. He avoids sugar although he occasionally has chocolate, as "you've got to have a treat somewhere along the line". His diabetes has never caused him to have a "hypo".

Eric has had three GPs in the 35 years or more that he has attended the same GP surgery. His current doctor lives nearby. When talking about his GP, he notes that hospital staff remarked that she must have been "on the ball" for spotting that he was deficient in vitamin D. He advises other people with diabetes to try and lose weight, although he has personally found this difficult.

www.healthtalk.org/peoples-experiences/long-term-conditions/multimorbidities/
eric#ixzz5XztAOSev

Madelon

Madelon is 93 and has "little strokes" and diabetes. She has been treated for stomach cancer and has had both knees replaced. She believes that her health problems are a result of being overweight. Madelon is a retired housewife, and her ethnic background is White.

Madelon's recurring strokes find her "talking a load of rubbish" and sometimes admitted to hospital. The effects of the strokes sometimes go away of their own accord. She has diabetes, which makes her tired. She takes a lot of prescription drugs, so many that she doesn't know "which is for which". Because she takes warfarin she has twice weekly trips to the GP surgery for blood tests. She believes this system is very well managed, but doesn't feel that she should be expected to make her own way to the surgery at her advanced age.

Madelon doesn't see her diabetes and strokes as being connected. She tries not to do anything too strenuous and "not to put myself under too much pressure". Her main issue is being released from hospital without social support:

"The only thing I've sort of had trouble with is when I've been in hospital, there don't seem to be much sort of care for when you come out and when you're on your own, but I think probably that's improved a bit because it's, you know, it's not very nice when you've been in hospital and then you come back to an empty house and got to cope with yourself".

Madelon thinks her GP is very good: "He's sort of listens and usually he's got a solution to whatever it is".

www.healthtalk.org/peoples-experiences/long-term-conditions/multimorbidities/
madelon#ixzz5XztxVDLn

Audrey

Audrey is 79, married with two children and is a retired office administrator. Audrey feels her sleep has deteriorated a lot in the last ten years. She rarely gets more than a few hours a night, and a really good night would be when Audrey sleeps for 4–5 hours. She would really like to sleep longer.

Audrey moved to their current home about ten years ago. She likes to keep active and belongs to several local groups. In particular, Audrey has found a lot of benefit from attending a group called S.M.I.L.E., So Much Improvement with a Little Exercise, and does feel she sleeps a bit better after going to these gentle exercise sessions.

Audrey feels her main sleeping problem is getting to sleep and often finds she tosses and turns for quite some time. She tries clearing her mind and imagining going through a long dark tunnel, but finds it very difficult to get to sleep. Occasionally, when she wakes up in the night and can't get back to sleep, Audrey will come downstairs and read the whole newspaper before going back to bed and trying to sleep again.

Sometimes Audrey finds she sleeps better on holiday than at home and wonders if this might be because she has been busier during the day. Audrey also finds that she sometimes dozes off whilst watching the news on the television after lunch. Audrey believes the deterioration in her sleep is largely because she is getting older, but also because she has quite a lot of pain in her legs and back.

www.healthtalk.org/peoples-experiences/later-life/sleep-problems-later-life/audrey-interview-39#ixzz5XzwbVQ3c

Index